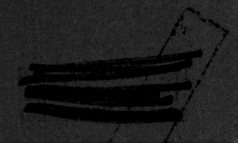

STROKES

and their
Prevention

STROKES

and their Prevention

How to Avoid High Blood Pressure and Hardening of the Arteries

Arthur Ancowitz, M.D.

 VAN NOSTRAND REINHOLD COMPANY

NEW YORK   CINCINNATI   TORONTO   LONDON   MELBOURNE

Van Nostrand Reinhold Company Regional Offices:
New York   Cincinnati   Chicago   Millbrae   Dallas

Van Nostrand Reinhold Company International Offices:
London   Toronto   Melbourne

Library of Congress Catalog Card Number: 74-13360
ISBN: 0-442-20330-6

Manufactured in the United States of America

Published by Van Nostrand Reinhold Company
450 West 33rd Street, New York, N.Y. 10001

Published simultaneously in Canada by Van Nostrand Reinhold Ltd.

15   14   13   12   11   10   9   8   7   6   5   4   3   2

Library of Congress Cataloging In Publication Data

Ancowitz, Arthur, 1925-
    Strokes and their prevention.

    Bibliography: p.
    1. Cerebrovascular disease. 2. Cerebrovascular
disease—Prevention. [DNLM: 1. Arteriosclerosis—
Prevention and control. 2. Cerebrovascular disorders—
Prevention and control. 3. Hypertension—Prevention
and control. WL355 A542s] I. Title.
RC388.5.A52   616.8'1   74-13360
ISBN 0-442-20330-6

DEDICATION

To the families who have had to cope with stroke, to those investigators whose work will prevent stroke, and to my Dad who suffered a stroke.

TABLE OF CONTENTS

PART TWO: STROKE AND PREVENTION

ACKNOWLEDGMENTS

To the countless scientists who strive to unravel the complicated threads that constitute the mysteries of hardening of the arteries and high blood pressure goes my deepest appreciation. It is unfortunate that they all cannot be individually acknowledged. They include investigators and teachers in the basic as well as the clinical sciences.

Dr. Howard Rusk was kind enough to review the manuscript. Dr. Joseph Cimino's introduction is gratefully appreciated. The author also wishes to acknowledge the encouragement of Drs. Albert Decker, Jerome Driesen, Robert Doud, Leonard Plaine, Arthur Schwartz, and M. J. Zweibach. Drs. Sidney Gross, I. Tarlov, and Frederic Weissman were kind enough to review the chapter on "anatomy of a stroke." Mrs. Sue Miller, Mr. George Fletcher, and Mrs. Mary Scott Welch were kind enough to offer their criticism.

Mrs. R. Granet and Mrs. M. Peets were of help in gathering references and source material. The assistance of Mrs. Ada DeVenuto, Mrs. Rose Rivera, Mrs. Elizabeth Sanchez, and Mrs. Rose Moravec is appreciated. Medical Reports Service was of help in the transcription of the manuscript.

To my family and to Mrs. Ellie Zweibach and Mrs. Sheila Drucker of my office staff go my appreciation for their forbearance and understanding in the preparation of this book. E. F. Cudlipp's contributions of professionalism, selflessness, and encouragement were vital to the author and this book.

INTRODUCTION

The American public has been underrated with respect to what it knows and understands medically. Better education and the media (that is, television) have elevated the public's knowledge and interest in medicine. Too many recent books, however, have enlarged on fads or promoted theories without a sound basis in scientific investigation, merely to catch the attention of a wide audience. At the same time that these books belittle the intelligence of the American public, they ignore the needs of all of us to be sensibly informed about such major killing diseases as heart disease, cancer, and stroke.

Although stroke ranks third as a killer, it is the single most expensive disease, costing some $1.2 billion a year —even before the costs of physicians' services and nursing homes and other nonhospitalized care are figured in.

There has been a pressing need for the public to become aware of the magnitude in numbers and the human tragedy that heart disease and stroke cause. Although a great deal has been written about heart disease, there has been little written for the general public about stroke.

This book tells the stroke story in a straightforward way. Honesty is not sacrificed for simplicity. Dr. Ancowitz's talents and experience as a teacher and clinician have been well utilized in presenting us with an informative and interesting book that does not skirt the issue. It does not spoon-feed us. It does not strike fear into us. It does give us understanding and hope. Wherever possible, he has presented the evidence on all sides of controversial questions without a loss of perspective. Entire books have been written on subjects to which only a chapter or two of this book have been devoted. Yet the reader will find these chapters refreshing and replete with informative material.

It is of paramount importance that the public be educated on the known risk factors in stroke and heart disease. Only through education can we reach the stroke-prone individual and encourage him to seek medical care in order to possibly prevent a stroke.

One of the major causes of stroke is high blood pressure. It has been called a widespread disease that we in Public Health must treat as vigorously as we would any epidemic. A minimum of 10 percent of the population has been estimated to have it. Millions of people are walking around, unaware that their blood pressure readings may be high enough to kill them. High blood pressure is not a disease with symptoms in its early stages. The victims feel well. Because of this, they don't seek the treatment that could save their lives.

For this reason, many cities have initiated high blood pressure (hypertensive) clinics and have started mass screening programs to identify those people with high blood pressure and advise them to see their physicians or to seek care at a clinic. In New York City, we are trying to locate these people through the many clinics operated by the Department of Health. We have been screening 10,000 people a month since May, 1972. We have found about 1,000 hypertensives a month. We have also been checking the blood pressure of high school students and youngsters applying for working papers. We have been surprised to find that one or two out of every 100 youngsters examined have some degree of high blood pressure and are considered hypertensive suspects. Regardless of the reason why anyone goes to these clinics, the person is checked for high blood pressure. If the blood pressure is elevated (many people are nervous simply from attending a clinic and their bood pressure may be elevated for this reason), the blood pressure is double checked. If it is still elevated upon recheck, the person is referred to his own physician or to one of the many public or voluntary clinics cooperating in the program.

Many other cities have set up their own programs, but there is still much that needs to be done: *First,* to identify the hypertensives who are highly stroke-prone and, *second,* to convince them to seek treatment and maintain treatment.

One reason for the emphasis on public programs to identify these people with high blood pressure is that it can be treated and treated successfully. Another reason is that through high blood pressure treatment and other medical advances, it has become possible to achieve a goal that has heretofore been elusive—some degree of prevention of heart disease and stroke. The profusion of knowledge presented by our hard-working scientific community can now be applied toward measures of prevention by the public at large. Scientific knowledge *per se* must be applied in order to be useful. However, in order to achieve this goal successfully, the American people must be informed. They usually respond if they understand and are aware of what they are dealing with.

It is toward this goal that this book is written. If we could apply even a small percentage of the funds spent today on the treatment of stroke toward the *prevention,* we would enhance our ability to prevent stroke.

At the same time, fear is not a weapon that should be used in telling the stroke story. Belief in the future of science as applied to preventive medicine gives us the hope that stroke is preventable as well as treatable. Dr. Ancowitz has tried to eliminate fear and provide hope through informing the public of scientific facts, presented in a readable and interesting way. Only in this manner can the public be informed and the dread specter of stroke be combatted.

JOSEPH CIMINO, M.D., M.P.H.
Commissioner of Health
New York City
January, 1974

PART ONE:

STROKE AND ITS CAUSES

What is stroke? Who gets strokes and why? What are the causes? What are the roles of hardening of the arteries and high blood pressure, diet and smoking?

These are only a few of the questions that this part raises. The answers, or as many of them as are now known, are to be found in the following pages.

CHAPTER I

WHAT IS STROKE?

Mrs. B.G., a woman in her 50's, was sitting anxiously across the desk from her physician. The doctor was trying to reassure and calm her fears. Her husband, the comptroller of a small construction firm that was having difficulties in meeting commitments because of union problems, had just had a stroke.

"But Doctor," she pressed nervously, "what do you mean by 'stroke'?"

"A stroke," he answered, "is a loss, either temporary or permanent, of functioning brain tissue. This loss of function results in a disability, which can take many forms, although the usual one is a loss of motor function on one side of the body, often accompanied by difficulty in speaking. The loss of motor function is paralysis; the difficulty in speaking is aphasia."

The answer didn't reassure her. All she could think of to ask was, "Does this mean that he is going to die?"

"Of course not. Strokes don't have to be fatal," the physician said. "In your husband's case, for example, the chances are good that he will recover." He didn't add that the recovery could include fringe disability.

Mrs. B.G. still didn't understand. She was thinking of her husband, whom she loved and had always tried to care for. "But Doctor, what caused it?"

"There could be many reasons," the physician said patiently. "Your husband is overweight. He smokes heavily. He's under a great deal of tension on his job.

He doesn't get enough exercise. He has high blood pressure. All these factors enter into why he had the stroke —although there may be other factors that we are just beginning to learn about."

"What can *you* do?" Mrs. B.G. asked.

"We're running tests to find out how much of the brain has been damaged," he told her. "Then, we'll know what we can do. But a lot depends on you."

"What can *I* do?" she asked in surprise.

"To begin with, support your husband all you can. Afterwards, he may need special care and devotion on your part to help him get dressed or eat. With time and attention, however, we have every hope that he will be able to return to work." The physician went on, "When he recovers, you can help prevent another stroke by making sure that he doesn't start smoking again, by keeping his weight down, ensuring he eats a prudent diet that's low in cholesterol and saturated fats. . . ."

This conversation, or one very like it, takes place in a physician's office every time a person has a stroke. These are the questions that relatives of every stroke victim want to ask, just as Mrs. B.G. did ask them. The answers are far from simple—there are, to begin with, different kinds of strokes. Some strike without warning, while others may have warning signs. While we know much about the causes of stroke, physicians cannot answer all the questions fully, and some questions may require more time to answer than a physician has or even than the patient's relative has.

The simple definition of what a stroke is, for example, may seem plausible to a physician and yet be difficult for a layman to grasp. At the same time, no stroke is easily described. There is not always a loss of motor function or speaking ability. Vision may be affected also or instead. So the results are often as hard to describe as what caused a stroke, although the word itself implies a sudden blow or attack, a kind of Pearl Harbor—with or without warning—in the brain.

An old medical term for stroke is "cerebrovascular accident." The term accident implies both prevention and the possibility that there are factors beyond a person's control. Take Pearl Harbor: at one level, there were warnings—intelligence sources warned that something was up. At another level, there was complete surprise. Strokes occur similarly.

Another medical term is "cerebrovascular insult." Certainly, there can be no greater "insult" to the brain than a stroke. Both terms, however, mean *stroke.*

The purpose of this book is to help us all understand the enormous frequency of stroke, its causes and effects, and most importantly, what can be done in the way of prevention.

One of the few positive effects of World War II and the Korean War was the explosion of knowledge, because of firm public support, in the field of rehabilitative medicine. To assist the injured veteran, our government wisely spent considerable funds to encourage the development of the science of rehabilitation medicine—physiatry. Under the influence of respected, dynamic personalities, such as Dr. Howard Rusk, the science of physiatry contributed not only to the care of our battlefield victims but also extended that knowledge to the stroke victim.

As vital as rehabilitation is, our attention must be turned toward prevention. The application of the latest and best knowledge and the encouragement of research will make possible a reduction in the death rate and the devastation caused by stroke.

These are the facts of stroke:

A stroke does not have to be fatal. It does not have to cost a person's life or ruin it because of physical disability or the loss of mental faculties, or even in the sense of financial ruin. Although more than 200,000 Americans will die of stroke this year, more than 2 million Americans who have had strokes are alive.

Strokes can be prevented. In the past, the emphasis has been on what happens *after* the stroke is completed, but we are starting to realize that we may be able to prevent stroke before it happens, if not in all of those 200,000 cases, in at least a significant number. If even one stroke is prevented, that is one life that will be spared a terrible cost in disability and money.

To understand prevention, we must first understand what a stroke is. The best way to understand this— what stroke is and what can be done to treat it—is to view a stroke through the lives of those who have had strokes. This will also help to show some of the ways in which stroke can be prevented.

The case of Mr. L.P. is one example.

L.P. as a child was more interested in art and drawing than he was in school and his academic studies, until he reached his teens. Then the teachers who had called him "dull" were forced to change their minds. He suddenly became aware of the sacrifices his father, a small businessman, was making for him to go to college. Science began to fascinate him more than drawing people's faces. Mathematics, physics, and chemistry filled his life even more completely than art ever had. By the time he was 25, he had made his first scientific discovery, dealing with the composition of crystals. He had also married the daughter of the dean at the college where he was teaching and working in the laboratory.

The pattern of his life was set—success followed success professionally. But what was he like as a person, and how did he treat success?

Those who worked with him, both in his role as professor and as scientist, had a hard time keeping up with him, intellectually and in the long hours that made up his day. L.P. was a perfectionist. He had a single-minded devotion to his work, combined with an intuitive "sixth sense" on whatever subject was foremost in his mind. He became angry only when his opinions and discoveries were attacked. According to a nephew, he had little sense of humor.

As a result of his work, he had made several important discoveries by the time he was 44. These improved both the standard of living and the efficiency of industry.

Next to his work, his only interest was his family—his wife and children and his parents, but personal tragedy added pressure to the tension of his work. His father died. He had barely recovered from his profound grief at this loss, when his 2-year-old daughter died. A year later, another daughter died. That same year, even greater pressures piled up when the college where he was then administrator and director of scientific studies erupted in student demonstrations. Although he continued to work in his laboratory at the college, he was relieved of his administrative duties. The result was that, instead of relaxing, he threw himself even more completely into his work.

One morning in October, he awakened at his usual time and had breakfast. Afterwards, he became aware of an uncomfortable tingling sensation in his left arm and leg. When he told his wife, she worried about it. She tried to get him to stay home and rest, despite his claim of "feeling fine now." His only compromise was to let her accompany him to the door of his laboratory to make sure he was all right. That evening, he went to bed early, only to have the tingling start again. Even worse, he had difficulty talking and his left leg was so heavy that he couldn't move it.

Mr. L.P. had had a stroke at 47, at the height of his productive years.

His wife stayed at his bedside all that first night, but it was morning before their doctor was called. The doctor did all that he could for Mr. L.P. Nevertheless, by evening the case seemed hopeless. Although L.P. never lost consciousness, he was drowsy, apathetic, and restless. In the morning, his mind was clear; yet despite the reassurances of his wife and friends, he was sure he was going to die. That week was a difficult one. By the end of it, he was recovered enough, though, to be able to dictate an outline for a new project to a student. Several weeks later, he returned to his laboratory.

His left side remained paralyzed for the rest of his life. Nineteen years later, when he was 66, he suffered a second stroke. This time his speech was seriously affected. Almost a year later, there was a third stroke. He didn't leave his room until his death eleven months later.

At the same time, during the nineteen years between his first and second strokes, he lived a fruitful and gratifying life. He overcame the handicap of having his left side paralyzed, his left forearm bent and contracted, the fingers clenched uselessly, and his left leg so stiff that walking was difficult. He went on to even greater discoveries in the field of science, moving into the area of medical research. His creativity and ability were never stoppered or thwarted.

L.P. was Louis Pasteur. Before his stroke, he evolved the method now known as Pasteurization. Afterwards he turned to immunization—first of sheep against anthrax, a disease that killed thousands of sheep yearly in France, and then of rabies, or hydrophobia, which afflicts animals and the human beings who are bitten by the "mad dogs." His wife, who had always written out his papers for him in those days before the typewriter, gave him more and more attention. Their two surviving children were grown and required little from her. They and especially Pasteur's son-in-law encouraged and helped Pasteur all they could, so that he never gave in to the sense of hopelessness that may accompany a stroke.

Mr. W.W. was a poet. His poetry was controversial for his time, so that although his genius had been recognized early by some critics, other critics condemned his work for being obscene. He had to fight for acceptance from the beginning, and when his work was published, the books didn't make enough money for him to enjoy a comfortable life. He was a sensitive man, always concerned with the suffering in the world around him. The money he did make often went to those he thought needed it more than he did.

He had a stroke when he was 39, from which he recovered completely. In his 40s, his life underwent a change. Into these, normally a man's most productive years, intruded a war. With the same wholehearted dedication that he put into his poetry, he threw himself into helping the wounded, going to hospitals and sitting long hours with the soldiers. The death he saw and the pain he shared wore him out. Even his poetry lost meaning for him. Through the help of friends, he was hired in a minor government position that provided him with a bare living. This security ended when he was fired because his superior decided that W.W.'s poetry, with its sexual overtones, made him a "poor risk." Again, friends rallied to his side and he was hired in another government position.

The war, his attempts to have his poetry published, the dissension of the jobs took their toll. Mr. W.W. complained of apathy and periods of dizziness for several years following his first stroke. He ignored these warning signals, and a second stroke confined him to his bed at the age of 55. This time he was partially paralyzed. Although the paralysis gradually receded, mental apathy set in. He admitted that his mind was affected too. If it had not been for his friends and family, Mr. W.W. could have become a permanent invalid. They helped him to lead a full, creative life. When he died at the age of 73, he died of tuberculosis—not of a stroke.

W.W. was Walt Whitman.

Whitman wrote *Leaves of Grass,* which was one of the most controversial poems of its day.

His treatment was typical of what a nineteenth century physician could do for a stroke patient. Bed rest was about it. More important were the encouragement of Whitman's mother and sister and several close friends, to whom his health and poetry were vitally important and who worked ceaselessly to cheer him up.

Pasteur, another man of the nineteenth century, had little else done for him when he had his first stroke. The exception was that the attending physician, one of the most famous of his day, bled Pasteur by applying sixteen leeches behind the scientist's ears. Other than that, it was bed rest.

Both men were proof that a stroke does not have to be fatal. Their biggest enemies were the feelings of apathy, despondency, and hopelessness that too often accompany a stroke, today as then. These two men could be called lucky, in that they were inspired by the love and devotion of those nearest to them.

Although Pasteur and Whitman might have been exceptional men, they were not exceptions. At that time, no one quite knew what a stroke was or how to treat it. They could be called lucky, too, in that they survived, regardless of the limited knowledge of the day.

It's a simplification to say that the strokes were not handicapping in the sense a poet or a scientist can manage to "create" with one hand. But what about a musician? Mr. G.F.H. was a cosmopolitan man of music. Although he was born in Germany, he composed and made Italian opera famous in England. He was reputed to be one of the greatest organists and harpsichordists of his day. A big, lusty man with an explosive temperament, he could turn around with a philanthropic generosity that was overwhelming. Four years after Mr. G.F.H. suffered a stroke, he wrote "The Messiah." He continued to compose for some eighteen years more, until his death in 1759.

Mr. G.F.H., of course, was George Frederick Handel.

The list of the famous who have had strokes is not confined to science or the arts—or to history. More than one President of the United States has suffered from symptoms of stroke or has died from stroke, according to Dr. Morris Fishbein, a dean of medical writing. These Presidents include John Quincy Adams, John Tyler, Millard Fillmore, Andrew Jackson, Rutherford Hayes, William Howard Taft, Woodrow Wilson, and Warren Harding, as well as Franklin D. Roosevelt. Interestingly enough, the three most famous, outstanding leaders, who led their countries during a long, hard war that changed the world, were the three participants of the Yalta Conference. Winston Churchill, Joseph Stalin, *and* Roosevelt all died from strokes.

Stroke, then, has no respect for position or genius, and it seems evident that stroke symptoms often appear in the productive years of a person's life. In short, anyone has the potential for having a stroke. That means you or me. The "anyone" includes women: Stroke does not respect sex—it is not a male chauvinist disease.

Miss P.N. is a beautiful and talented actress, whose roles have run the gamut from glamour to character parts, one of which won her an Oscar. When the stroke hit, she was happily married and devoted to her husband, a successful writer, and their children. A few years before the stroke, she and her husband had known near tragedy when their toddler son had been badly injured in an automobile accident. He had recovered from the bodily injuries, but the brain damage lingered, requiring numerous operations and expensive therapy. As a result, her career had suffered. Yet, at the time of her stroke, her life had seemed to be settling into a happier pattern. The little boy was doing well with therapy; she was pregnant.

The near tragedy of her son may have been a "blessing in disguise"—possibly it saved her life. The boy had a tendency to go into convulsions after the accident because of his head injury. When P.N. had her stroke, her husband recognized the symptoms of brain involvement right away and called a neurosurgeon friend. P.N. was rushed to the intensive care unit of a nearby hospital. Thanks to the care of her doctors and the knowledge that physicians have gained about stroke since the days of Handel, Pasteur, and Whitman, P.N. survived.

Her battle for life was not over. She spent weeks in a coma under intensive care; specialists examined her and prescribed medication and treatment according to their specialties; her husband devotedly repeated over and over to her his belief that she would recover completely. Her own determination and the love and devotion of friends helped her and her doctors to win the battle. After she left the hospital, she needed a leg brace to walk, her face was still partially paralyzed, and she was starting speech therapy in her struggle to put words and meaning together. She won her battle so successfully that within two years she made her first speech in public and resumed acting. She also bore her third child, who was normal and healthy.

P.N. is Patricia Neal.

Modern medicine helped save her life. Advances in rehabilitative therapy enabled her to recover completely enough to return to acting. But plain, old-fashioned hard work was as important as anything else. Few who saw her before and have seen her since in movies or on television can detect any trace of the stroke that almost killed her.

Stroke, then, is not necessarily fatal.

Stroke does not need to have the tragic after-effects so often associated with it, but treatment should be started as early as possible and pursued intensively.

Stroke does not mean that a person can no longer work in the same profession or create as competitively as before. *Complete recovery is possible.* Stroke is not a hopeless disease.

Despite these facts, stroke has been a much-neglected disease for many years. Professional people have shown little interest in it, and the public—until the start of the last decade—generally accepted stroke with resignation. Until a few years ago, moreover, many in the health profession considered that patients with a stroke had a feeling of utter hopelessness and helplessness and *were* hopeless and helpless. Their difficulties in speaking and communicating made it hard for them to express their feelings and wishes, so they were left alone. It wasn't even too long ago that many stroke victims, as a result, were hidden in back beds in hospital wards, where relatively little was done for them, other than giving them custodial care. The house staffs of the best hospitals considered the stroke patient a "crock"—one whose disease was commonplace and not esoteric enough to merit more active treatment.

What makes stroke especially tragic is the strain and actual cost of treatment. Hospitalization, rehabilitation, and other expenses have been estimated at about $25,000. The cost can be even higher, since all too often the family is deprived of a provider or homemaker.

If the victim is unable to function effectively, he thus is deprived of reaping the rewards of a lifetime.

A stroke can affect a family in other ways, too.

For example, the illness can have a psychological effect on the family. The constant need for emotional support on the part of the stroke victim means that other members of the family may have to sacrifice their own emotional needs. There is also the physical disability, the help a person may need in eating, walking, or caring for other life functions, and the difficulty in communicating those needs.

But this is what happens after the stroke has occurred. What happened to cause the stroke in the first place? Why are some people affected in one way and other people in other ways? These are the questions most often asked of the attending physician, and the explanation at the beginning of the chapter—simple as it is—only scrapes the surface of answering them or describing the complexities of stroke.

There are three principle causes of stroke: (1) ischemia, (2) hemorrhage, and (3) emboli. These are called *vascular strokes. Vascular* means that the stroke originates in blood vessels.

Ischemia means a lack of oxygen carried via the circulation to a particular part of the body. This can result from a narrowing of the artery or a blockage of the artery carrying blood-rich oxygen and glucose. The blockage is called a *thrombosis;* the narrowing is called *stenosis.* In the case of the circulation to the brain, oxygen and glucose are necessary for the life of the nerve cells. Depending on the area of the brain involved, the right or left side of the body may be affected, along with difficulties in vision and speech. For example, if the right side of the brain is affected by the stroke, it will be the left side of the body that suffers a loss of function. If the left side of the brain is affected, the right side of the body has a loss of function.

Pasteur was extremely lucky when he had his first stroke in that, being right-handed, the paralysis occurred on his left side. Also in Pasteur's case, a relatively small, localized area of the brain had been involved. The larger the area, the greater the involvement, as with Patricia Neal.

Although paralysis, temporary or permanent, almost always results from a stroke, the involvement can also include speech and mental abilities. A person may be paralyzed, unable to talk or to connect words with meaning, with much greater involvement. Diagram A shows the particular area of the brain that controls these various functions, with the area of damage linked to the function it controls.

Ischemic strokes may be due to many causes, such as hardening of the arteries *(atherosclerosis)*, in which the circumference of the arteries gradually becomes smaller, thus decreasing the supply of blood being circulated through some areas of the brain. A factor in the formation of atherosclerosis is the blood fats. Studies have shown that excessive cholesterol, a fatlike material found in certain foods as well as in the human body, forms plaques (deposits or patches) that build up on the walls of the arteries, thus narrowing them and not permitting adequate blood flow. (See Chapter III.)

One kind of ischemic stroke is the thrombotic stroke. A thrombosis is a clot, in this case one occurring in an artery and obstructing the blood flow to the brain. Again, depending on where the brain tissue is injured by the interrupted flow of blood and oxygen and glucose, the particular function controlled by that part of the brain will be affected, with paralysis, loss of speech, body-function control, and so on.

Ischemic strokes are sometimes preceded by warning

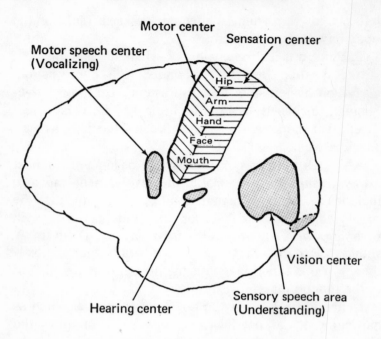

FIG. 1   SEVERAL IMPORTANT CENTERS IN THE BRAIN
CONTROLLING SPECIFIC FUNCTIONS
(SIDE VIEW)

signs. If these had been known in Pasteur's and Whitman's day, the warnings might have helped prevent
their strokes or, at least, have warned them to slow
down. These signs include short periods of paralysis,
numbness, or dizziness, or the tingling that Pasteur had
noticed before his first stroke. Understanding what
causes stroke can be a form of prevention if the *signals*
are heeded.

Thrombotic stroke is the type that has been tied to
birth control pills. Any woman who takes, or has taken,
the pill receives with her prescription a booklet or in-
struction sheet warning her about reactions. One reaction may be blood clots occasionally forming in the
blood vessels of her legs and pelvis. These clots can

break loose and lodge in the lung. More significant concerning stroke is that the clots can also form in the brain.

For these reasons, women who use the pill are carefully advised by their physicians of the possible side effects. Needless to say, however, millions of women throughout the world have found birth control pills reliable and safe.

Pasteur's stroke was a classic in other ways—such as the time of day it occurred. Although a stroke may happen at any time of day, it most frequently occurs in the morning after a night's sleep. The theory of why strokes occur at night is that blood pressure decreases when one is asleep. In patients who go on to get strokes at night, it is felt that the pressure of blood in the circulation to the brain might have been inadequate. This type of stroke carries the best chance of useful survival, depending on which blood vessels or area of the brain is involved. *Ischemic or thrombotic strokes injure only a specific area of the brain supplied by a specific blood vessel and, in so doing, cause specific functional impairment.*

The second and next most common type of stroke is a stroke caused by a brain, or cerebral, hemorrhage. *Cerebral hemorrhage* (sometimes called *apoplexy*) can be defined briefly as bleeding within the brain as a result of blood vessels that burst, impairing the circulation of the blood and its vital oxygen and glucose to that part of the brain. As with any stroke, the result is a loss of function or functions controlled by the brain tissue affected. Massive hemorrhage can destroy large areas on *both* sides of the brain, causing rapid loss of consciousness and death. It was this type of cerebral hemorrhage that caused the death of President Franklin Roosevelt.

More limited cerebral hemorrhages usually carry a proportionately better outlook or prognosis. The two major causes of cerebral hemorrhage are high blood pressure and abnormalities of blood vessels. Since the discovery of effective anti-high blood pressure drugs, the prevention of cerebral hemorrhage is a distinct possibility. If it does happen, however, it can be treated more effectively.

Embolic stroke is the third kind of stroke. This stroke is due to small emboli or clots, which may form on the heart valve or on the inner surface of the heart and travel to the brain. Although other kinds of stroke generally occur at the periphery (the ends of the blood-distribution system), this stroke strikes at the "heart" of the circulatory system. It may be the result of rheumatic heart disease, a heart attack, or infection of the heart valves. At the same time, this form of stroke is becoming increasingly rare since there is a lowered incidence of rheumatic fever and an increased use of anticlotting drugs. The classic clinical work of Dr. Irving Wright with the anticlotting drugs has contributed to our better understanding of this type of stroke.

In summary, there are three kinds of stroke: Ischemic (or thrombotic), cerebral hemorrhage, and embolic strokes. Understanding what form a stroke can take can help remove some of the apprehension caused by such medical terms as *cerebral infarction*. Being aware of the warning signs can help the stroke victim to get the immediate attention that will save his life; the sooner medical help is sought, the greater chance there is for complete recovery.

Since thrombotic strokes do often occur at night, let us consider the case of Mr. D.J. as an example of what happens and what forces modern medicine has at hand to help a stroke victim get the latest care, both in diagnosis and treatment. Mr. D.J. could be called a typical stroke case. He is an average man, with average talents and abilities, no one famous. He had recently had his

60th birthday. He had been healthy all his life and was looking forward to retirement in a few years, when he and his wife planned to move to Florida.

He went to bed one night as usual. During the day and the evening before, he had felt fine. The next morning when he awakened, his speech was slurred and he found, like Pasteur, that he could move one arm and one leg only with difficulty. With Mr. D.J., it was his right side. In other words, the left side of his brain had been affected by the stroke.

His wife immediately called their family doctor, who needed only to hear the symptoms to order hospitalization. In the hospital, Mr. D.J. was placed in the intensive care unit, a room especially designed to monitor all the body's vital signs—heart, blood pressure, and even brain waves. D.J.'s breathing was labored; his heartbeat slow but regular. By then he was semiconscious.

The difference between what little could be done in the nineteenth century and what can be done today is the difference between night and day, the horse and buggy and the modern sports car, and the ultimate in the latest medical resources and techniques. At Mr. D.J.'s command, so to speak, were as many as forty-eight diversely and highly trained men and women who formed a team that could organize at a moment's notice to treat the stroke victim in order to limit the nerve damage. In Mr. D.J.'s case, that might mean being able to return to work, finishing out his productive years at his job, and retiring with full pension, able to enjoy his retirement. He need not be forced to retire to a bed or a wheelchair, subsisting on whatever pension his company plan and social security entitled him to at his age.

The concept of the stroke team is relatively new. The stroke team is composed of, or can enlist, many special-

ists, including an internist, a neurologist, a neurosurgeon, a stroke nurse, and a physical therapist, supported by a computer programmer, a statistical clerk,
and other nursing assistants. The information collected
is constantly monitored, reviewed, and edited to provide
the most accurate information. Each member of the
team becomes more effective as a result of the coopera-
tion, so that planning, treatment, and rehabilitation are
better coordinated.

Mr. D.J. was treated by a stroke team consisting of
his own physician and others, such as a neurologist who
assessed the extent of the damage and performed a spinal tap. The neurosurgeon was available for consultation
in the event that the stroke was caused by a surgically
correctable process. The physiatrist, a specialist in rehabilitative medicine, outlined a program of progressive
therapy for Mr. D.J. A speech therapist saw him and
applied the latest techniques to evaluate and treat his
language dysfunction. He had numerous blood tests, as
well as tests to access his neurological status, all performed by various specialists and laboratory assistants.
Included among the tests done were the brain-wave test
(electroencephalogram), a radioactive brain scan, and
skull X rays. Mr. J.'s diet was expertly adapted by the
dietician to be consistent with his swallowing ability and
his caloric needs.

The nursing part of the team was responsible for su-
pervising the feeding and skin care and the general
comfort of Mr. D.J. His encouragement to improve
often came from a friendly voice or a kind smile from
one of his nurses. The nonprofessional people, the people who do the menial tasks, are the ones the patient
often remembers the best. The attendants, people who
clean up, and secretarial staffs are all important
members of the team.

Although some of the details of treatment for stroke

patients such as Mr. D.J. are often routine, therapy on the whole requires the utmost in ingenuity and adaptability. The overall treatment and therapy can never be routine, predetermined, or automated. Such cookbook therapy is outmoded for strokes.

Under the care of the stroke team, Mr. D.J. had available all of the resources and talents one finds in good general hospitals. These were ready and available to serve his needs. But Mr. D.J.'s recovery was not solely due to the stroke team. The patient's recovery is the product not only of what is done *to* the patient but also of what the patient himself is capable of doing and what *he* himself wants to *do*. It was due, in large measure, to the *desire* of Mr. D.J. to recover and to the hard work that he, his family, and the team performed.

Knowing what a stroke is, is only a start. If anyone can have a stroke, is there any way of locating the people who may be more prone to stroke?

We think so. In the subsequent chapters, we will learn of some of the warning signs of stroke and some of the predisposing conditions that may lead to stroke.

CHAPTER II

WHO GETS STROKES

Just about anyone can have a stroke, and stroke *is* the third largest killer of Americans after heart disease and cancer. But why did those particular 200,000 or more Americans die of stroke last year? Why did any one of those people have a stroke, instead of someone else?

Let's put it this way. Every year 7 million automobiles roll off our assembly lines. Most are mechanically perfect. Yet, standardized and ideal as the assembly line is, every year a few cars slip through with faults that make them *accident-prone*. Some faults may not be serious in themselves—one untightened bolt may cause a complaint by rattling, but two untightened bolts may combine to create an accident-prone condition, needing only the right moment or circumstance for the accident to happen.

An accident-prone car can be an engineer's nightmare. He has to search for answers to such questions as: How can this condition be corrected? Why did it happen and why, to that model? What can we do to prevent the same thing from happening in the future?

The answers may involve a massive call-in of a particular model, even though only a few cars may be accident-prone. Yet the call-in is necessary because car manufacturers want to identify accident-prone cars *before* the accident.

When it comes to our bodies, the problem is both similar and different. Our bodies are so complex that medical science has not yet been able to identify all the accident- or stroke-prone trouble spots. Even though one human body is similar to another in many respects of physiology, there are individual differences. *We* do not come off assembly lines—unless we're identical twins. At the same time, there are certain individual factors and other factors in combination that predispose some people to stroke, just as mechanical errors can predispose some cars to accidents. The human factors leading to stroke make up what is called the *stroke-prone profile*.

Studies made during the past couple of decades have begun to bring out theories and consolidate ideas about phenomena occurring in the body that often precede a stroke. It seems apparent that certain physical conditions or diseases have some relationship to stroke, making those people with them more predisposed than others to having a stroke. Identifying who those stroke-prone individuals are is the first step in stroke prevention.

Since men make cars, the errors are equally man-made and can be located with certainty. The difficulty with stroke is that, with few exceptions, there is controversy concerning just about all the factors that may contribute to, or have some effect on, stroke. We think one of these exceptions is hardening of the arteries, or generalized atherosclerosis. There is also little doubt that high blood pressure or hypertension contributes to the development of a stroke-prone condition. It is felt that high blood pressure may have a direct connection to the deaths of 250,000 or more Americans each year by severely straining their cardiovascular systems. The heart and the arteries that serve all the vital organs, including the brain, suffer. Less well defined is why deaths due to high blood pressure occur among blacks at more than twice the rate they occur among whites: 58.4 per 100,000 for blacks, as opposed to 27.1 per 100,000 for the white population, according to Department of Health, Education, and Welfare statistics.

Because of the importance of both atherosclerosis and hypertension to stroke, both are mentioned now but are treated more extensively in separate chapters later on. In the meantime, these are only two of the human phenomena that are thought to have a bearing on stroke. Personal habits, like smoking, as well as genetics, in which certain physical weaknesses or conditions are inherited, and even other diseases seemingly—to the layman—unrelated to stroke may play a part in identifying individuals who tend to be prone to stroke.

Many of these factors played a part in one of the most outstanding studies made of cardiovascular disease. This study was carried out over a period of years in Framingham, Massachusetts. In 1949, when it started, Framingham's population of 28,000 represented a microcosm of the American population as a whole—ethnically, economically, and sociologically. The town itself, 21 miles outside the city of Boston, consisted of factories surrounded by pleasant suburbs. More than 5,000 men and women between 30 and 62, who were healthy and free of heart disease, volunteered for the study. Their medical histories included a history of any parents or grandparents who had had cardiovascular problems. The crux of the study involved complete physical examinations and laboratory tests every two years. Among the tests were ones for blood-cholesterol levels, electrocardiograms, tests for diabetes, and lung capacity. Also considered was cigarette smoking. In short, the study covered just about every factor that has ever been thought to have any relationship to cardiovascular disease.

The *full scope* of cardiovascular disease was what the National Heart Institute wanted to find out about. Since the heart is a pump that distributes blood through the body, such conditions as atherosclerosis and high blood pressure have a bearing on the heart's ability to provide that service. Thus any controversy over cholesterol and atherosclerosis, for instance, will be as controversial in causing heart attacks as it is for stroke.

The difference between the two—heart disease and stroke—is relative. They might be called "kissing cousins." In stroke it is the arteries of the brain that have "hardened" rather than the arteries serving the heart. Although this is a simplification, it does serve to show how what we learn about the heart helps us to understand stroke, too. As a result of the Framingham study, therefore, we have been able to understand *all* cardiovascular disease better, including stroke.

There is one "hard fact" we can start with: By the end of 14 years, 135 strokes had occurred: 70 in women and 65 in men. Of these, 63 percent were thrombotic (ischemic) in origin, 22 percent were due to cerebral hemorrhage, and 15 percent were due to emboli.

The habits and medical records of the 135 stroke victims were analyzed. Through these comprehensive analyses, the picture of a stroke-prone individual began to take form. Some of the factors involved have been mentioned, and some are considered to be important enough to be discussed separately. All are, nevertheless, a part of the stroke-prone profile.

The order in which they are listed is arbitrary, with no attempt to list them in order of importance. Any one factor or condition may not be enough to predispose a person toward having a stroke, but a combination is probably significant. Most of the factors take into account conditions that can—and should—be treated.

Developing the Stroke-Prone Profile

1. *Sex and Aging.* Traditionally, sex and aging are supposed to play a part in any stroke-prone profile. They are important—who ever thought we could and would be tinkering with sex and aging? It would seem that sex and the process of aging are immutable, but not so! Attempts to modify and deter the aging process are being investigated. The influence of sex hormones to modify atherosclerosis is also being studied.

According to statistics, men have more strokes than women. Although men have a tendency to have strokes at a younger age and women at an older one, the age when both are most stroke-prone is the same—about the age of 60. In hospitalized stroke patients, the ratio of strokes occurring in males is about two strokes to one in women, in the U.S. white population, and approximately three to two in the U.S. black population. The reasons for the difference are not clear. Contributing factors, such as heart disease, smoking, and lung disease, tend to appear earlier in the male and probably play some role in the sex difference.

One line of research has been to try to prove that men have more strokes, in general, than women because female hormones protect women longer than male hormones do men. Attempts to prevent strokes in men by giving them weak female hormones, however, have been unrewarding. Although most females who have strokes have them when they cease making their own hormones, the hormone theory does have a strike against it. In recent years, the rising incidence of stroke in women of child-bearing age who are taking birth control pills has been related to the female hormones, notably estrogen. Since statistical evidence shows that women taking oral contraceptives do tend to have abnormal clotting of the blood, there is some suggestive data associating the pill with a risk factor in stroke.

A recent study made by twelve collaborating university medical centers found that women using an oral contraceptive ran a risk of having a stroke that was nine times greater than for women not on the pill. It emphasized, however, that the increased risk, large as it sounds, is small because women of child-bearing age rarely have stroke. Present oral contraceptives with a very small amount of estrogen decreases even this risk.

An added finding suggested a possible relationship between the pill and cigarette smoking. Of the women who did have strokes, a large proportion smoked cigarettes regularly. Women who have pill-related clotting but not strokes, also tend to be smokers. The reason is that cigarettes increase the tendency of platelets, one of three kinds of cells in the blood, to aggregate or clot.

These findings bear out the results of previous studies, in that women who have thromboemboli in any part of the body or have had any episodes suggesting a transient cerebral or retinal attack (vision difficulties), as well as women with hypertension or severe migraine, are better off using some other form of contraceptive than an oral contraceptive. Every woman on an oral contraceptive should inform her physician of any out-of-the-ordinary symptoms or side effects.

As far as aging is concerned, statistics tell the story. What they indicate is a warning for stroke prevention care to start early, because stroke occurs in the most productive years of life. In general, 14 percent of all strokes occur in persons under the age of 50; 45 percent occur in persons under 59; and 83 percent happen before the age of 69.

2. *Transient Ischemic Attacks (TIA)*—These are the warning signals of stroke. Professor P.G. is a 52-year-old, hard-working, intense professor of medicine at one of our eastern medical schools. He arrived late to class one morning for his weekly lecture to his fourth-

year medical students. During the course of the lecture, his students noticed that the professor's speech became slurred and unintelligible. He couldn't turn the pages of his lecture notes with his right hand. He appeared in good control of himself, but he sat down and rested for a few moments before resuming his lecture.

Professor P.G. told his students that he had just experienced a transient ischemic attack. Actually, what he had noticed himself was numbness and weakness in his right hand as he turned his lecture notes. He had also suffered some dizziness and visual difficulties. Within minutes, all of his symptoms disappeared, and the professor led his students in a discussion of TIA. Subsequently, he had a thorough physical examination, including X rays of the arteries of his neck and brain. It was found that he had a significant narrowing in the left carotid artery in his neck. Corrective surgery was successful in averting a stroke, so that Professor P.G. was returned to health. His outlook is excellent.

TIA are statistically the most important factor in the stroke-prone profile. The most conservative estimate is that 20 out of every 100 persons who have these attacks will have a lethal or incapacitating stroke (a completed stroke) within a period of five years, if they are left *untreated*. Other estimates of stroke run as high as 70 out of every 100 persons who have had TIA. At the Mayo Clinic, where several series of cases were followed for five years after their first TIA, about 35 percent of the patients had strokes later.

These warning signs, therefore, should be to us like a red flag is to a bull. They should arouse us to action.

Medically, a transient ischemic attack is a temporary stroke occurring in a localized area of the brain. The attacks or episodes may last from 2 to 15 minutes, although an occasional episode may continue for as long as 24 hours. Between attacks, the person is completely normal. They generally leave no persistent aftereffects. The person is normal after the attack. Sometimes there is no way to distinguish clearly between a TIA and a neurological deficit that may be happening for various other reasons, since the symptoms may be similar. The important point to remember is that any episode with these symptoms needs prompt attention and treatment. Once a TIA is diagnosed and treated, the person may avert permanent damage and disability. (Also see Chapter VIII.)

3. *Obesity.* There is no clear evidence of a direct relationship between obesity *per se* and the increased risk of stroke—but obesity *is* often accompanied by an increase in blood pressure. Both weight and heightened blood pressure do add to the load put on the heart, so that the risk of heart disease increases. In addition, obesity usually leads to a decrease in the person's general mobility. Thus a person who is overweight is wise to lose weight to decrease the possibility of cardiovascular disease.

Moderate obesity, from 10 to 20 percent over the ideal weight tables, was not a factor in cardiovascular disease, according to the Framingham studies—*unless* there were also high levels of cholesterol in the blood. At the same time, insurance actuary tables do link overweight with earlier death from a variety of causes, including cardiovascular disease. Lean is better than fat for a number of reasons—and that also goes for the food we eat.

4. *Hypertension.* Agreement is practically unanimous on the importance of high blood pressure as a risk factor in stroke. The Veterans Administration Cooperative study showed that the probability of *death* from heart failure and stroke was lowered by decreasing the blood pressure. In addition, as far as stroke was concerned, people with lower blood pressures had fewer

strokes. Sustained hypertension, on the other hand, definitely increased their susceptibility to ischemic stroke with an infarction (death of brain tissue) or hemorrhage within the brain.

The Framingham study is supported by statistical evidence from other sources, showing that the *incidence* of stroke, usually cerebral hemorrhage, is higher in untreated or inadequately treated hypertensive patients than in persons with normal blood pressure and persons with hypertension that has been adequately treated. (See Chapter IV.) Since effective methods of treating hypertension have become available, mortality from cerebral hemorrhage has begun to decrease.

5. *Congestive Heart Failure, Enlargement of the Heart, and Electrocardiographic Abnormalities.* Heart disease as suggested by an enlargement of the heart or certain electrocardiographic abnormalities is strikingly related to increased risk of stroke. Certain types of irregular beats of the heart predispose a person to strokes caused by emboli (traveling plugs). Appropriate treatment of the existing heart disease reduces the person's risk of stroke and so does the use of anticlotting medications.

6. *Hypercholesterolemia.* This simply means an increased amount of cholesterol in the blood. Cholesterol is a blood fat that is found in humans and in all other animals. Beef, lamb, pork, organ fats, and certain types of seafood are especially rich in cholesterol and can boost human blood cholesterol levels.

Although hypercholesterolemia has been linked to atherosclerosis as a risk factor, its importance as a cause of stroke is not unanimously accepted. The Framingham study did associate it strongly with an increased risk of stroke in persons under 50. After the age of 50, the researchers could find little relationship between cholesterol and stroke. Just as hypertension alone does have some bearing on stroke, however, so does cholesterol—and elevated blood cholesterol *and* hypertension together are considered to be more serious than either abnormality by itself.

It is another case of lean being safer than fat. Lean meats, skim milk, and certain vegetable-oil margarines raise cholesterol levels less than do well-marbled prime steak, whole milk, and butter.

A rare condition that runs in some families, called *hyperlipidemia* and meaning high blood-fat levels, is associated with a high incidence of heart disease and stroke. Early diagnosis and treatment can avert trouble. Hypercholesterolemia, however, is not necessarily a family trait, except that the family that eats together can raise their cholesterol levels together.

7. *Diabetes Mellitus.* A great deal has been written about the relationship between hardening of the arteries and diabetes. Diabetes accelerates atherosclerosis. At some hospitals, the incidence of diabetes in patients admitted with a diagnosis of cerebral infarction (stroke) has been reported to be as high as 30 percent. Again, the Framingham study data show clearly that the risk of stroke is increased by diabetes, even if the person has only a moderate elevation of the fasting blood sugar. (Increased blood sugar, after a person has fasted—not eaten—for a standard period of time, is an index of diabetes. Blood sugar normally rises after eating.) In persons with both diabetes and hypertension, as with high cholesterol and hypertension, the risk of stroke is even greater. In the case of diabetes and hypertension, it is six times greater than in nondiabetics with normal blood pressure.

There are no really significant observations available to show whether precise control of diabetes will reduce the risk of stroke in diabetics. Nevertheless, diabetes should always be treated and controlled to avoid possible complications. In fact, a person with diabetes couldn't do better than to have his diabetes monitored regularly by his physician.

8. *Polycythemia and Other Hematological (Blood) Disorders.* Blood is composed of three different cellular elements in a watery solution. The cells are the red cells, white cells, and platelets. An increase above normal in all three types of cells is seen in a condition known as *polycythemia* (*poly,* many; *cythemia,* blood cells). Normally, blood flows like a watery solution through the arteries. In polycythemia, it flows like a thick oil without its usual freedom of movement.

Changes in the constituents of the blood can affect circulation in the brain, so polycythemia plays a real part in the stroke-prone profile. As the blood increases in viscosity or thickness, the possibility of a stroke increases.

Other hematological disorders associated with stroke include certain other types of high red-cell counts, such as that seen in chronic pulmonary disease, where there is an increased concentration of carbon dioxide and decreased oxygen supplies in the blood, thus depriving the brain of the oxygen it needs. There are a number of conditions that are also factors in stroke in which the blood does not clot properly or in which the tendency to stop bleeding is lost. Conditions such as hemophilia and conditions where there is a lack of a variety of clotting factors in the blood predispose these persons to stroke.

9. *Hyperuracemia. Hyperuracemia* means an elevation of uric acid in the blood. It is associated with gout. From time to time, a relationship between gout and hardening of the arteries is suggested. Some patients with stroke do have high serum levels of uric acid.

As with diabetes, gout should not be left untreated. Gout is one of the few diseases, when treated adequately, whose effects are practically completely reversible.

10. *Cigarette Smoking.* Statistically, cigarette smoking is a risk factor in stroke. In the Framingham study, persons who smoked cigarettes seemed to run excessive risks for all types of cardiovascular disease and atherosclerosis (Chapter III). This was particularly demonstrated in men, by the numbers of male cigarette smokers who had stroke. Other studies have shown similar links—and similar results.

In short, whatever the relationship between cigarette smoking and stroke, the effects of cigarettes on atherosclerosis are ample enough reasons for *both* men *and* women to stop smoking.

11. *Emotional Stimulation.* Constant emotional upset and tension may lead to deleterious effects on our hearts, arteries, and nervous system. It is a good bet that we can all profit by a minimum of upsets. This factor, as with hypercholesterolemia, atherosclerosis, and high blood pressure, seems important enough that it, too, will be treated in greater detail later on.

12. *Cardiac Arrhythmias.* Irregularity of heart beats (cardiac arrhythmia) can cause a decrease in the blood supply to the brain and may induce transient ischemic attacks or more permanent effects. A particular type of heartbeat irregularity known as auricular or atrial fibrillation can often give rise to emboli (plugs that emanate from the heart), which may travel to the brain.

What happens in and to the heart affects the brain because of the effect on the cerebral blood flow. A large number of TIA, for example, occur at the very outset of the various cardiac arrhythmias. But if the arrhythmias can be prevented, so can a majority of the TIA. Some irregularity can be corrected through medications, others by means of a pacemaker that regulates the rhythmic beat of the heart.

13. *Genetics.* If we could have our "druthers," we'd

pick parents who died at a very old age, whose families were free of heart disease, diabetes, high blood pressure, and stroke. We might even prefer that they originally came from one of those areas of the world, such as a remote part of Russia or Pakistan, where people are said to live to be well over 100, still carrying on the business of their everyday life, hale, hearty, and stroke-free.

How important is genetics in the stroke-prone profile? And what role does environment play?

Cigarette smoking, the kinds of food we eat, the water we drink, the type of life we lead with its stress and tension are a part of the environment. We do know that they may, and probably do, have some relationship to stroke, but environmental factors don't explain entirely why some people have strokes and some don't, why some people live to an advanced age with no sign of cardiovascular disease and others who die young have severe changes in their arteries. The inability to find complete answers in environment is one reason for looking to genetics. Genetics determines whether we are born male or female, the color of our hair and skin and eyes, and also certain physical and chemical abnormalities.

Family studies tend to bear out a genetic link to coronary heart disease. One of these was carried out in England, where the male relatives of victims of ischemic heart disease were followed up. Those closest in blood relationships, the first-degree relatives, had a risk of death from the same heart disease that was five times greater than the population as a whole.

Genetic studies with human beings have one handicap—the average life span is so long that it's impossible to follow families through the generations necessary to trace genetic trait. Animals are another matter. Squirrel monkeys have been used for studying the genetics of blood cholesterol. Although all were being fed the same diet, some developed high blood cholesterol levels; others showed little change; still others had a blood cholesterol level that fell between the two groups. The monkeys were bred within the same groups. Invariably, the progeny of those highly susceptible developed the same high cholesterol levels in their blood, with the offspring of the other two groups following the same patterns as their parents. Yet all the monkeys were being fed the same diet. Genetics did play a role in how the monkeys made use of their diet. It undoubtedly plays a role in humans.

Some types of hyperlipidemia (discussed in 6 above) definitely run in families. This type of hyperlipidemia is detectable in infancy. It responds to diet, which reduces the serum cholesterol level in the blood, thus reducing the chances of premature cardiovascular disease. Undetected and untreated by either diet or medication, this abnormality can result in premature heart attacks.

Genetic factors may have an influence on hypertension. Although this theory is controversial, statistically the death rate due to high blood pressure for blacks is more than twice that for whites, as mentioned earlier. (See Chapter IV.) The search for the genetic connection has been carried to Africa, where studies have tended to be concentrated in East Africa. This part of Africa is rural, and many of the people still follow the customs of their forefathers. As far as hypertension goes, there is little of it. Recently, however, researchers have studied West Africa, which is where the majority of American blacks originally came from. There is more hypertension as the people move from farming villages into urbanized areas. The race link to genetics, therefore, is inconclusive, with the environment, stress, and the tensions of modern life playing some undefined kind of role.

14. *Miscellaneous Factors.* Various other conditions may have a bearing on stroke. For example, arterial diseases associated with certain types of syphilis can lead to stroke. This factor, although very rare, does not have the broad impact on stroke as do some of the other factors listed above.

Who, Then, Is Not Apt to Have a Stroke?

All of the various factors listed in this chapter enter into a prestroke profile and stroke prevention. Obviously, few people are going to have all these diseases or conditions, but anyone who has any, or any combination, of them, most physicians feel, is more stroke prone than a person who has none.

The importance of the factors above is that most can be treated, if the condition is detected, thus reducing the risk of stroke. It is good preventive medicine, as well as good sense, never to let any correctable conditions go untreated. The sooner they are detected and treated, the better chances a person has for leading a healthy and fruitful life. Granted, some of these conditions may be treated more easily, but it cannot be repeated often enough that *most can be treated successfully.*

We mentioned accident-prone cars at the beginning of the chapter, and we raised this question: Why does the assembly line slip up on only *some* cars? We could also ask why some cars, regardless of what happens to the other cars, always seem to roll off in perfect condition. The answer to both questions is that, although man is capable of making mistakes, he is also capable of righting his mistakes.

When it comes to stroke, we've answered the question of why some people seem to get strokes—they have certain conditions or diseases or live in such a way (the way they eat, smoking) that they predispose themselves to stroke. At the same time, just as a car can have its accident-prone conditions corrected, most of these conditions in man can be treated by a physician and corrected by the person himself.

We know that the less accident-prone car is the one that has even the smallest bolt tightened. By the same analogy, we know that the person who is the least stroke-prone is the one who has the fewest conditions predisposing him to stroke. It stands to reason, then, that you are *less* apt to have a stroke if:

1. You are a woman of child-bearing age, not taking the "pill."
2. You are close to average weight for your height and age, according to ideal weight tables. You are lean.
3. Your blood pressure is within normal bounds.
4. You have no history of heart disease or are being adequately treated for heart disease.
5. Your blood fats are normal.
6. You eat a lean diet, avoiding cholesterol-rich foods and saturated fats.
7. You don't smoke or have given up cigarette smoking.
8. You receive adequate treatment for associated diseases.
9. You avoid undue stress or undue emotional tension, and you exercise regularly.
10. You have a kind of genetic protection, by having parents and grandparents who lived to a ripe old age. Unfortunately, there's nothing much you can do about this factor, since you can't pick your parents.

CHAPTER III

HARDENING OF THE ARTERIES
AND STROKES

A new car is a wonderful piece of machinery. Every part has been tooled and polished to perform a certain function. Fuel lines carry gasoline inside smoothly finished "tubes" to provide power to the engine, enabling it to move the car forward at the speed you desire (and sometimes even faster). Oil from the crankcase keeps the engine lubricated and running evenly, without friction. The car's nervous system, the wiring, is pliable. Within a matter of months, aging starts, aside from any built-in obsolescence. Metal rusts, pipes clog, dirt and inefficiently burned fuel particles gum parts.

A car can be repaired—just about any part can be replaced. If the repairs are expensive, the car can be traded in for a new model. A consumer has the same choice for any machine or any appliance, from an electric toaster to a computer, even though a computer is about the most sophisticated and "human" of all machines. Machines are man-made, and what man makes man can replace with a new model each year.

The human body is a unique machine. When it ages, it may creak—but it won't rattle. Parts may be "traded in," the outstanding example being kidney transplants. But we have to live with our own bodies, and we can neither replace nor trade in one body for a "newer model." Nor can we stop the aging process, although we tend to take far better care of the car or appliance we keep only a few years than of the bodies we have for a lifetime.

Ironically, people understand more about what happens inside a car than what is happening inside their bodies. A clogged fuel line in a car is simpler to grasp (the car is hard to start, sluggish in responding to the foot on the accelerator) than a clogged or clogging artery. This is what virtually happens in hardening of the arteries, or atherosclerosis. Yet, hardening of the arteries is as inevitable in our bodies as aging is to a car. Both are a kind of built-in obsolescence.

The fact that sooner or later everyone will have some atherosclerosis is as certain as it is predictable. As a part of the human aging process, it is as natural as the fact that a car's fuel lines will clog with dirt. But just as the dirt doesn't become dangerous in a car until it plugs the fuel lines, atherosclerosis doesn't become a disease until it affects the arteries of an important organ—the heart, kidneys, or brain. Even so, despite this inevitability, we are studying ways to *de*celerate the progress of atherosclerosis and to treat it more effectively. There's hope.

Individual and mass screening programs using what are called provocative tests can detect atherosclerotic disease that is present, even if the symptoms are not apparent. Early atherosclerosis of the coronary (heart) arteries or the cerebral (brain) arteries may be without telltale symptoms or signs. It is *subclinical*—that is, without symptoms—and this subclinical disease may be ushered in without warning in the form of sudden death due to a heart attack or stroke. About 20 percent of the people who die of heart attacks had no prior symptoms or suggestion of heart trouble.

The purpose of provocative tests is to head off these heart attacks and strokes. Exercise tolerance tests are used to bring out abnormal electrocardiographic changes in persons who are otherwise considered to be healthy. The person being tested will be tested at rest and then doing exercise. Abnormal findings may suggest atherosclerotic changes in the coronary arteries, and these changes may respond to a treatment program.

What Is Hardening of the Arteries?

Hardening of the arteries or *atherosclerosis* or *arteriosclerosis* is a ubiquitous and sneaky disease. It can and does affect just about everyone, everywhere, at any time—and all the time. The process, when arteries begin to harden, starts when we are quite young, in the main artery of the body, called the aorta, where it does no harm. This hardening of the arteries is seen in the arteries of children as yellow streaks. These streaks of fat are a natural phenomenon occurring in virtually all people and animals.

As we get older, the tempo of atherosclerosis lags until the third decade of life, at which time the fat causing the streaks accumulates increasingly in the arteries and affects specific, critical arteries. These critical arteries are the arteries to the heart (coronary arteries), the arteries to the brain (cerebral arteries), and the arteries to the kidneys (renal arteries). During the development of this slow, steady process, the person is quite well. There is no pain, no discomfort attached to the relentless development of atherosclerosis.

The yellow or fatty streak progresses to a plaque, which severely limits the diameter of medium and small-size arteries, much in the way rust and dirt can narrow a fuel line in a car. The atherosclerotic plaque, however, contains fat and other components that the body calls upon to surround the fat.

At the stage where the plaque narrows the artery, a clot or thrombus may form in the artery. The formation of this clot prevents blood and its vital oxygen from reaching the tissue involved.

ARTERIES (LIFELINES) AND THEIR OBSTRUCTIONS

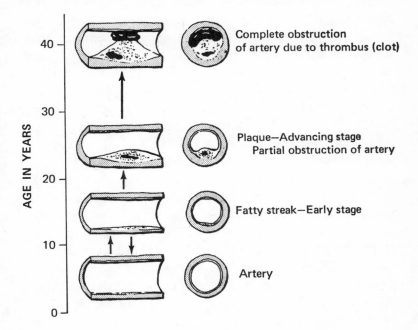

FIG. 2 DEVELOPMENT OF ATHEROSCLEROSIS AND ARTERIAL OBSTRUCTION.

Death of the tissue results. In the case of the heart, the *coronary thrombosis* causes a *myocardial infarction* —a heart attack. In the case of the brain, the *cerebral thrombosis* causes a *cerebral infarction*—a stroke.

A plaque is formed around fat. Cholesterol, triglycerides, and phospholipids are the three major fats in the blood. Phospholipids are mainly concerned with the transport of fats to the liver and to the fatty parts of our body. Triglycerides are simple fat and are found wherever our bodies are padded or rounded. Our favorite actresses are well endowed in the right places with triglycerides. Too much triglycerides in the *blood,* however, is something we can do without.

The same is true of cholesterol.

Whenever the blood has too much cholesterol or triglycerides, the technical term, *hyperlipidemia,* may be used. The special importance of hyperlipidemia is that it may predispose the person to atherosclerosis, heart disease, and stroke. Because cholesterol and triglycerides (like most fats) aren't soluble, a transport system is achieved by their hooking up with proteins in the blood. The resultant molecules are called lipoproteins. They are graded according to the size of the molecules and their density.

The low density lipoprotein is the lipoprotein most usually related to heart disease, when it occurs in excess. It is the low density (LD) lipoprotein that gets trapped in the wall of the artery. The fat is thought to enter the artery wall by infiltration. This means that, as the blood flows through the arteries, the fat within the blood penetrates the wall of the artery and stays there. Although the arteries are muscular tubes through which blood flows without "leaking," fat filters through, with only the LD lipoprotein being caught.

Since the measurement of lipoproteins is not as yet routine, valuable information can be obtained by measuring the serum cholesterol and serum triglycerides. Usually when both are elevated, the risk for atherosclerotic heart disease is increased. The brilliant work of Dr. D. S. Fredrickson has contributed to much of our knowledge about blood fats and their consequences.

In a system of distensible tubes, such as our beautifully ordered vascular (blood vessel) system, the theories of fluid dynamics are obeyed. Changes in blood pressure and turbulence help determine where the plaque forms—where the disease strikes in the arteries. The hydraulic effects of pressure changes probably account for where atherosclerotic plaques will form in this system. Accordingly, plaque formations will, and do, occur where there is narrowing, splitting, or branching of the arteries. It is at these points that LD lipoproteins gain easier access to the artery walls and that plaque formation occurs to a great extent.

Because atherosclerosis has a varying tempo—some people get it sooner than others—all of the factors in our environment are looked at as possibilities to modify its rate. Then, too, because some arteries in one part of the body may suffer more advanced changes than other arteries, associated disease factors are also suspected.

There may be factors modifying the advance of hardening of the arteries, too. Some of these factors are sex, age, race, diet, nutritional state, body build, hormones, diabetes, high blood pressure, occupation, emotional stress, and smoking.

What Causes Hardening of the Arteries?

Many research laboratories around the world are involved in the study of atherosclerosis. Particularly of interest to us is:

1. What accounts for the acceleration of hardening of the arteries in some people and not in others?
2. Is it reversible? Can atherosclerosis, once present, be modified or helped to disappear?

An interesting study using the Rhesus monkey has been done by Doctors Taylor, Cox, and others investigating the effect of diet on hardening of the arteries. The findings point up some of the causes of hardening of the arteries, as well as providing some clues about what happens to the arteries in the aging process. The investigators have found these facts:

1. Supplementing the standard primate diet with butterfat and cholesterol crystals causes severe elevation of fat in the blood and severe atherosclerosis, with a buildup of plaques and consequent narrowing of the arteries.
2. Marked acceleration of the atherosclerotic proc-

ess occurs if a 50-50 mixture of coconut oil and butterfat is used to supplement the cholesterol-enriched ration. These are *saturated fats*.

3. There were severe changes if the animals were fed peanut oil, in that existing plaques were aggravated.

4. In animals fed corn oil, there was little evidence of atherosclerosis. Corn oil is an *unsaturated* or *polyunsaturated fat*.

A supplemented primate diet is one thing—what about the typical American diet? An experiment in the laboratory of Dr. Robert W. Wissler involved Rhesus monkeys that were fed a typical American diet. Although they weren't served a plate of bacon and eggs for breakfast or a juicy steak for dinner, the ingredients were mixed into a paste and fed to the animals. (The way food is prepared does not affect basic nutrients. You may add fat to fry eggs, for example, but you don't change the nutrients. Protein is protein, although vitamins may be "cooked out" of vegetables.) Other monkeys were fed the "prudent" diet recommended by the American Heart Association. This diet is designed to reduce the intake of saturated fats and cholesterol.

The results indicated that the animals on the typical American diet had high blood fat levels and showed atherosclerotic changes in the arteries. In contrast, little serum fat changes and atherosclerosis were seen in animals on the prudent diet.

Some people argue that we humans are hardly monkeys in our behavior, makeup, and intelligence, while other people suggest that primates (man and monkeys) have too many biological similarities to be ignored. There are differences—if monkeys haven't invented a computer, they also haven't invented guns or made war. Apart from intelligence and behavior, there *are* the biological similarities, with the strong experimental evidence that links atherosclerosis to diet—in particular, certain types of fat and cholesterol. If we don't ignore it, and it seems too strong for that, we can all benefit from these observations.

If hardening of the arteries can be experimentally induced, for example, there is also substantial experimental evidence that atherosclerosis can be reversed through dietary modification, use of hormones, and cholesterol-lowering drugs. These reversal experiments suggest that atherosclerosis may not be the relentless, inevitable process it was once thought to be, and intelligent attempts at further reversal in the light of our present knowledge are certainly called for.

The matter of hardening of the arteries and diet does have another side of the coin.

Intrigued by the fact that atherosclerosis has a predilection for obstructing arteries where they fork, branch, split, or curve, Dr. Meyer Texon has devoted himself for many years to studying this phenomenon. Dr. Texon feels that damage done to the arteries obeys the laws of hydrodynamics. The sites of branching and curving of arteries are the sites where the greatest stress is placed on the inner wall of the artery. This stress is related to the speed of flow of the blood—the faster the flow, the greater the stress. The greater the stress, the more the artery is injured and the greater is the amount of resulting atherosclerosis. Atherosclerosis will occur irrespective of blood cholesterol or blood fat levels.

Reports of studies on groups of peoples eating a high-fat diet also suggest that the matter of the hardening of the arteries may not be so simple. Somali camel herdsmen subsist on a diet of about five quarts of camel's milk per day. Again in East Africa, the Masai—a traditional warrior tribe noted for being tall, thin, and graceful—drink a great deal of milk. Both groups are said to have a low rate of hardening of the arteries, but these observations must be tempered by the very high death rate due to infectious and other diseases. The average age of death in many of the developing countries is quite low, perhaps not giving hardening of the arteries enough time to develop.

Coronary heart disease has been shown to be relatively uncommon in Africans as compared to many Caucasian groups. However, the South African Bantu and their white compatriots are seemingly equally affected by hardening of the arteries going to the brain. In Nigeria, lesions of hardening of the arteries to the brain are rare as compared to American blacks in Alabama and among Bantus. High blood pressure was common in all three groups, but the blood cholesterol level was lower in the African groups. How far the differences in cultural characteristics and way of life contribute to these observed differences is unknown.

Alaskan Eskimos are similar to the Masai and Samburu in eating a diet of high cholesterol. They, however, have high blood cholesterol levels; but existing hardening of the arteries seems less severe, rarely resulting in complications. One explanation in their case is that their dietary pattern alters in a yearly pattern of high and low cholesterol. These alternating periods may, in some way, help the Eskimos to handle the cholesterol.

An interesting, and perhaps more pertinent, study was performed comparing Benedictine and Trappist monks. The Trappists do not eat fish, meat, eggs, or butter. The Benedictines do. The Benedictines have a higher average blood cholesterol level than the Trappists. No striking differences were observed with respect to the effects of atherosclerosis in both groups, although both groups seemed to have less heart disease than the general population.

Although the evidence regarding fat, diet, and hardening of the arteries is mixed, the prevailing weight of evidence indicates that a low-fat, calorically adequate diet will do us no harm and very probably a great deal of good.

Cholesterol and Saturated Fats

Cholesterol, a fatty substance that is odorless and tasteless, is found in all animals, as well as animal products. It is manufactured in the body, which uses it to manufacture hormones and bile acids. Cholesterol, therefore, is essential to life.

Once manufactured, cholesterol is carried throughout the body by lipoproteins in the blood. This blood cholesterol level can be influenced by dietary cholesterol in egg yolks, meats, butterfat, shellfish, and organ meats. Almost all foods, in fact, except for vegetables, which contain no cholesterol, have or may have an effect. Another influence on blood cholesterol are dietary fats, which are divided into three groups: saturated, unsaturated, and monosaturated fats.

Saturated fats are the fats (such as marbled fat in steak) found in cholesterol-rich foods and in coconut oil. These fats are solid at room temperatures, the only exception being coconut oil. Unsaturated or polyunsaturated fats are the liquid oils, the oils made from vegetables and including corn oil, cottonseed oil, and safflower oil. Monosaturated oils (peanut and olive oil) fall between the saturated and unsaturated oils.

These fats have properties that tend to affect the cholesterol level in the body. Saturated fats elevate the blood cholesterol level, while unsaturated fats tend to make it go down. Monosaturated fats have no effect on the cholesterol level, but it is reported that they may aggravate the atherosclerotic lesions already formed.

How much cholesterol *in the blood* is too much?

The national cooperative Pooling Project (of which the Framingham Study was one part) came up with some statistics. As the cholesterol level of the men in the study increased from less than 175 milligrams to 249, the number of first major heart attacks increased in proportion to the rise in the cholesterol level. At cholesterol levels of 250 to 274 milligrams, the number of first major heart attacks almost doubled over the lower levels. At levels of more than 300 milligrams, these events zoomed dramatically—to more than three times the number of those persons with a blood cholesterol level of less than 175. The number of coronary heart disease deaths also increased somewhat proportionately, but not to the level of the first major heart attacks.

On this basis, how much cholesterol *in the diet* is too much?

The standard American breakfast of bacon and eggs contains more than twice what it is felt the entire cholesterol intake for 24 hours should be, with the eggs alone accounting for about 500 milligrams of cholesterol, not counting what is in the bacon or the butter on the toast or the saturated fats. The American Heart Association, the American Medical Association, and other federal, state, and local health organizations, therefore, agree that most Americans need to change their eating habits. This doesn't mean going on a diet in the sense that most Americans diet, by counting calories. It does mean following a prudent diet, such as that in Chapter X, and playing it safe for the present rather than being sorry later on.

Does your blood cholesterol level have to be high in order for you to go on a prudent-type diet? Not at all. We think that everyone, by and large, can benefit from such a diet.

Diet is not the only method of controlling cholesterol levels. For one thing, in some people a prudent diet has no effect on reducing the levels of fat in the blood. For another, not all people can eat the prudent diet. A person with certain gastrointestinal disorders (for example, diverticulitis, or colitis) may not be able to eat the raw vegetables or even some of the cooked ones that are the backbone of a low-cholesterol diet. These people may need cholesterol-lowering drugs.

One drug is clofibrate (Atromid-S). In a five-year study of 1,400 airlines ground personnel, one group took clofibrate daily, while the other took placebos. Among the older men, those taking the placebos had three and a half times the number of heart attacks as did those taking the drug. Among the younger men, those not taking the drug had eight times as many heart attacks as those not using it. The results of this study may not be entirely due to the effect of the medicine on serum cholesterol. Other effects of the medicine may be important, too. It may prevent clotting in some obscure manner.

What We Know—What Is Being Done

Much of what we have learned about hardening of the arteries has come through autopsies. Until the Korean War in the early 1950s, it was thought that hardening of the arteries didn't happen at all until a person reached middle or old age. During the war, it was learned that hardening of the arteries in the arteries leading to the heart was appreciable in almost eight out of ten soldiers in their late teens and early twenties. These were soldiers who had been killed in battle and were healthy in all outward respects. It was considered that the development of atherosclerosis was as normal in them as it would be in other healthy men of their age.

The International Atherosclerosis Project (IAP), which investigated hardening of the arteries among people in several different countries, has made similar findings. In addition, it has found that coronary atherosclerosis is generally more extensive in men than in women. The maxim about women being the weaker sex doesn't seem to hold true when it comes to athero-sclerosis.

Although autopsies may be useful in helping us to understand what happens in hardening of the arteries and when it starts, they are hardly possible or practicable as a means of determining who has hardening of the arteries and how far the process has progressed. The early diagnosis of hardening of the arteries is difficult. The process goes on and on for years without symptoms. We study its possible effects when it is quiescent by provocative tests—stress tests.

Usually hardening of the arteries is harmless until it involves the arteries of the heart, brain, or kidney to the point that sufficient blood cannot be brought to those vital organs.

Take the case of Mr. A.B.C.

Mr. A.B.C. is a 42-year-old executive vice-president of a large building supply firm. This company has a policy of having stress tests performed on those in line for the presidency. Although his routine electrocardiogram was normal, Mr. A.B.C.'s exercise electrocardiogram was abnormal. He had a thorough physical examination, which revealed that he had hypertension and a high serum cholesterol. These two factors, in combination with the abnormal electrocardiogram, were indications of possible trouble ahead from hardening of the arteries. After suitable treatment, including Mr. A.B.C.'s following a prudent diet, he had another stress test. This time, the results were normal, and he was elected to the presidency of his company.

Despite the seemingly obvious value of the test, a serious problem with it is the reluctance of many organized groups to accept the exercise electrocardiogram findings as the basis for disqualifying a person from sensitive positions. The tests, for example, have been suggested for airline pilots but they have objected. As the tests become more refined, they will meet with fewer objections. Studies are now being made by Dr. S. E. Epstein of the National Heart and Lung Institute on refining and making the exercise test more specific.

Efforts are also being made to meet objections to changing our diet. The threat that steak and bacon and eggs may be eliminated from the American diet is being taken so seriously that researchers are starting to investigate a different angle of the problem: modifying the animals providing the meat we eat, rather than solely the effect of the meat on human beings. This line of research concerns the saturated fat in meat. A feed company in Idaho is experimenting with new feeds that it hopes will produce animal products with a high content of polyunsaturated fat.

We can't wait for this possibility, attractive as it sounds. In the meantime, we have to rely on the prudent diet and medications to control fat levels in the blood. Waiting for a warning or symptom of hardening of the arteries can be fatal, since the first warning for some people may be their last. It may be a heart attack or stroke. Following a prudent diet may be insurance against either one.

The odds are in your favor if you start now.

CHAPTER IV

HIGH BLOOD PRESSURE AND STROKE

At least 20 million Americans—10 percent of the total population—have high blood pressure. High blood pressure is epidemic. No other physical condition presents so many problems, is so puzzling, and is so potentially dangerous, since high blood pressure is related to a variety of diseases, including stroke. More than one study has closely correlated elevated blood pressure to the risk of heart or stroke death.

Accelerated hardening of the arteries has been called a disease of affluence because of its association with the cholesterol and saturated fats found in steak, lobster, butter, and other "rich" foods. High blood pressure or hypertension can be called "everyman's" disease. Many of those 20 million don't know they have it, and those who know may not care, regardless of the proof showing that high blood pressure increases a person's susceptibility to heart trouble, stroke, and kidney disease.

High blood pressure, unlike hardening of the arteries, has no affinity for one sex or the other. It is a constitutional equal right for both men and women. In young adults, after the juvenile period, the frequency of high blood pressure is greater in men than in women. In the middle years, this tendency evens out. In older people, the incidence of high blood pressure is greater in women.

Less equality exists in race. As mentioned earlier, high blood pressure strikes black communities harder than white ones, with estimates ranging from a low of one in seven blacks having high blood pressure to four in ten. What's more, it develops at an earlier age, frequently in the teens, and is more severe in blacks. The death rate from hypertension among black men between 25 and 44 years of age is fifteen times higher than among white men in the same age group. For black women, the death rate is seventeen times higher than for white women. According to Department of Health, Education, and Welfare statistics, more than 13,500 blacks die every year as a result of hypertension—this is a rate of 58.4 per 100,000 for blacks as compared to 27.1 per 100,000 for whites.

Both statistics indicate the magnitude of the problem, which is the reason for quoting them. Experienced clinicians who deal almost exclusively with high blood pressure tend to agree, however, that the disease is more prevalent *and* more difficult to treat in blacks than in whites.

Because so many "everymen" and "everywomen" have high blood pressure—without knowing it—mass screening programs have been devised to reach people and call attention to blood pressure. These are similar to earlier screening programs for tuberculosis and programs for polio and measles vaccinations that have all but caused those diseases to disappear. A weekend program in New Orleans attracted some 30,000 people, more than one-third of whom had high blood pressure. If these figures are borne out by future surveys, that estimate of 10 percent of Americans having high blood pressure may have to be completely revised—upward. In the meantime, in order to understand *high* blood pressure, what is blood pressure?

Blood Pressure and Its Meaning

Blood pressure itself is easily defined. It is simply the amount of force required by that unique muscular organ, the heart, to circulate blood through the series of tubes that make up the arterial system of the body. It is measured by the familiar rubber cuff that your doctor fastens around your arm and pumps up with a rubber bulb. What the gauge is measuring is the systolic and diastolic blood pressure.

The heart, to pump the blood, contracts. The contraction forces blood through the arteries. Systolic blood pressure is the pressure exerted by the contraction. When the heart and arteries relax, diastolic blood pressure is produced.

An average blood pressure in adults is approximately 120 systolic over 80 diastolic, written as 120/80, and referred to as 120 over 80. More simply, this means that arterial blood pressure should, at its height, drive a column of mercury up a tube to a distance of no more than 120 millimeters (about 4.7 inches). The column, at its lowest, should then fall to 80 millimeters (3.2 inches). These are the measurements taken by the blood pressure machine known as a *sphygmomanometer*.

If the blood pressure is elevated above levels such as 140/90, a middle-aged adult is said to have hypertension, or high blood pressure. Any elevation of blood pressure above 140/90, however, is not necessarily abnormal. Blood pressure can vary above the average for any number of reasons—including a person's being under some degree of tension, if for no other reason than being in a doctor's office. This tension, of itself, may induce a slightly elevated blood pressure, so that a physician may ask the person to return for subsequent blood pressure checks. Only after you are relatively relaxed can a true blood pressure reading be obtained. Some persons are so hypersensitive to the blood pressure cuff that they only have to have the cuff around their arms and—zoom—the blood pressure mounts dramatically. This kind of hyperreactive state is not necessarily an indication of high blood pressure disease.

Sometimes it's suggested that patients with high blood pressure take their own blood pressure at home in order to get a record of their blood pressure readings. This isn't as simple as it sounds.

Mr. J. H. is a school psychologist with high blood pressure. Because he worried about his blood pressure, he learned how to take it himself, investing in a blood pressure cuff and stethoscope. He took his blood pressure several times a week, and every time it was high. He called his physician, who arranged for the psychologist to come to the office. His doctor took the man's blood pressure, and it was normal. Despite the reassurance, Mr. J. H. returned home and took his blood pressure himself. Again it was high.

Mr. J. H., at ease in his physician's office, became so nervous taking his own blood pressure that it rose dramatically. Again, this kind of hyperreactive state doesn't mean that a person has high blood pressure disease.

High blood pressure must be distinguished from *high blood pressure disease.* Not all conditions associated with high blood pressure are abnormal or a disease state. The blood pressure is normally elevated when a person engages in strenuous physical activity; for example, running a race. There are emotional reasons, as well, for the elevation of blood pressure. These include being alarmed, very apprehensive, or very frightened.

To distinguish between high blood pressure caused by physical activity or emotional tension and high blood pressure disease can sometimes present problems. After a suitable period of rest and relaxation, however, the blood pressure should not be elevated in normal people. If the blood pressure is elevated when a person is rested and relaxed, an abnormal condition exists.

High blood pressure that is sustained at all times will produce a variety of disease states, unless corrected. What happens to this person whose blood pressure is continuously elevated? Several things *can* occur: His heart may be enlarged and fail due to the additional work required; his kidneys may be affected; his arteries may suffer advanced hardening of the arteries—and he may suffer a stroke.

Sustained elevation of blood pressure is not only a sign, it is a disease as well. Elevation of the systolic blood pressure, systolic hypertension, has a separate significance from elevation of the diastolic blood pressure.

Systolic hypertension may be caused by certain rare diseases of the heart, by aortic atherosclerosis, and by thyroid overactivity. We think it is less directly involved in stroke than diastolic hypertension.

Diastolic hypertension is a sustained elevation of the lower figure in the blood-pressure reading; that is, above 90, as in *150/100*. The 100 indicates diastolic hypertension, which may be caused by a large number of different conditions. It is diastolic hypertension, moreover, that is related to heart disease, stroke, and kidney disease. If there is no known underlying cause or disease that can be held responsible for the elevated blood pressure, persons with diastolic hypertension have what may be called by any one of three terms: primary hypertension, essential hypertension, or hypertension of unknown origin. These are synonymous, and which one is used may depend on your physician. If there is a known cause, the high blood pressure is called secondary hypertension.

Secondary Hypertension

Although secondary hypertension accounts for only 10 to 15 percent of all hyptertension, it is always considered by the family physician before he treats the high blood pressure. He will check reasons for it, such as kidney disease, since glomerulonephritis, pyelonephritis, and congenital kidney disorders can be causes of secondary hypertension. Treating these conditions may take care of the high blood pressure, but they must, in any case, be treated to prevent further complications.

The adrenal glands, located astride the kidneys, may also be a cause of secondary hypertension. The adrenals manufacture a hormone called aldosterone that helps the kidneys regulate the body's salt and water levels. Overproduction of aldosterone, which may be caused by a tumor in the adrenal glands, can result in high blood pressure. Another tumor of the adrenal gland can cause intermittent or sustained high blood pressure, too. This rare tumor is called a pheochromocytoma. This tumor pours out adrenalin and an adrenalin relative called noradrenalin into the bloodstream, causing high blood pressure. Removing the tumor causing overproduction of aldosterone or the pheochromocytoma can completely reverse the course of this type of high blood pressure disease and return the blood pressure to normal. Still another cause of high blood pressure is due to the excess production of a cortisone-like hormone from the adrenal gland.

Another cause of high blood pressure is coarctation of the aorta. In this condition, there is a narrowing or pinching of the main artery of the body—the aorta— resulting in high blood pressure in the upper extremities and low blood pressure in the lower extremities. It is one of the principal causes of high blood pressure in the young and, if detected early enough, is completely correctable. What happens is that in coarctation, the aorta is pinched after it leaves the heart so that blood is forced upwards, elevating the blood pressure there. Since not enough blood is moving through the stricture, the blood pressure in the lower areas of the body will be correspondingly lowered.

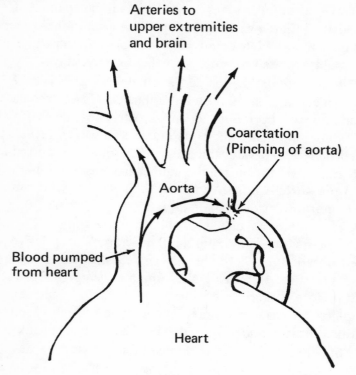

Arteries to
upper extremities
and brain

Coarctation
(Pinching of aorta)

Aorta

Blood pumped
from heart

Heart

FIG. 3   COARCTATION (PINCHING) OF THE AORTA

Although there are other causes of secondary hypertension, these examples are enough to show why high blood pressure should never be left untreated. If no secondary conditions causing hypertension are found after a thorough examination, the person is considered to have primary, or essential, hypertension. This is the case of about 85 percent of those 20 million persons who have high blood pressure.

Primary or Essential Hypertension

Primary hypertension or sustained high blood pressure of unknown cause needs to be treated early and

vigorously to prevent complications that can result—
including heart disease, stroke, and kidney disease.
These are three good reasons for the mass screening
programs that have been devised to find those people
with high blood pressure. Elliot L. Richardson, when
he was Secretary of Health, Education, and Welfare,
said that high blood pressure plays an indirect, if still
ill-defined, role "in the more than one-and-a-half million heart attacks and strokes that Americans suffer
each year. Nearly half of these heart-attack and stroke
victims die, and the majority of those who don't die are
paralyzed or severely restricted in activity."

Although primary hypertension does not have a
direct cause, there are several factors that have been associated with it. Obesity is one.

Fat may even contribute to a falsely elevated blood
pressure, since some elevations of blood pressure are
due to the excess fat around a person's arm. This fat
acts like a cushion, causing a false high blood pressure
reading. Other elevations of blood pressure because of
obesity are not so easily explained away, although the
single most important factor in high blood pressure that
is open to environmental and personal influence is
weight reduction. The relationship between obesity and
hypertension seems definite—as weight rises, so does
blood pressure. As weight falls, so does blood pressure,
indicating that some forms of hypertension are reversible in some instances by merely losing weight.

Losing weight is admittedly a terribly difficult and
even frustrating task for both the patient and the physician. Dieting, fad dieting, the use and abuse of medications in an attempt to lose weight have all been attempted with very little, if any, permanent success. The most
important and effective considerations to any program
of successful weight reduction are the patient's psychological background and motivation. These have been

used with great success by Weight Watchers as well as clubs, community groups, hospital groups, and the family physician who provides the backbone of the therapy. The aim is to create new food habits, since most obesity is simply the result of overeating and bad food habits.

The laws of thermodynamics cannot be repealed. If you eat 1,000 calories, you have to burn up 1,000 calories to avoid gaining weight. If you eat 1,000 calories and you burn 2,000 calories, you will lose weight. If you eat 1,000 calories and you burn 500 calories, your body will store the excess nutrient and you will gain weight. Exercise may seem one way to help burn off the calories.

A pound of body fat is the equivalent of 3,500 calories. A person who walks an hour a day burns up at least 300 calories. As long as the food intake isn't increased to make up these calories, a walk of an hour a day for a year could mean a loss of 20 to 25 pounds. But for most people the only—and the best—way to lose weight is to lose their bad food habit of overeating.

Several other factors play important roles in hypertension.

Great excesses of *salt* in the diet are not far from obesity in raising blood pressure. As closely as can be measured, the average American diet contains about 15 grams of salt per day—and this amount is probably rising every year because of the content of salt in commercially prepared "convenience" foods. Although a strict, low-salt diet has become archaic as a method of treating high blood pressure because of the excellence of medications, there is still a school of thought that utilizes very rigid salt restriction in lowering high blood pressure.

The heavy-handed use of salt in the American diet may reach back to infancy, according to some experts, especially because of the popularity of prepared baby foods, all of which contain salt. Although nutritionists argue that humans do need a certain amount of salt, the feeling in some quarters is that baby foods may be salted more to the mothers' tastes than to the babies', whose taste buds are less discriminating. Leaving the salt out may not affect a child's appetite, but—this argument goes—the mother, tasting the food, would add the salt herself.

Cigarette smoking is also a factor in hypertension. Cigarette smokers run an additional risk of cardiovascular mortality if they have a blood pressure reading in the upper ranges, above 140/90, than do nonsmokers. As a result of the data from the Framingham study, the risk of sustained high blood pressure is increased by cigarette smoking. The number of first major coronary events increased rapidly as diastolic blood pressure rose above 85 to 94 milligrams of mercury. Diastolic pressure of more than 105 nearly quadrupled the risk of a major coronary event over a pressure of less than 75. These two—high blood pressure and cigarette smoking in tandem—may be more dangerous to health than a high blood cholesterol by itself.

Tension or stress plays an as yet undefined role in high blood pressure. We do know that tension can cause a temporary elevation of normal blood pressure readings. The University of California Medical Center at San Francisco asked some high blood pressure patients to cooperate in a study. Outfitted with portable recorders to note their blood pressure, they performed their normal, daily duties, keeping a diary of what they did and what happened. The diaries were coordinated with the blood pressure readings. Under tension or stress, blood pressure did rise. One patient's blood pressure became elevated, for example, every time he used the phone to persuade the person on the other end to do something.

There are many kinds of tension. In one study, men facing unemployment had elevated blood pressure during the period when their job loss was anticipated. After they found new jobs, there was a significant reduction in the readings. It was considered that the psychological tensions of unemployment and job changes caused the elevation of the blood pressure.

The inner conflicts of accepting things as they are versus combative inner drives and desires are considered a possible psychological basis of high blood pressure. In addition, resultant suppressed anger enters into the inner turmoil, which may feed the fuel causing psychologically based hypertension.

There are several theories about tension. One is that if emotions are held back, kept inside, long enough, the temporary rise in blood pressure may not be dissipated and may, in time, become permanent. This is what some researchers feel may be the reason behind the high rate of hypertension in black communities, especially ghetto areas. The economic pressures, the danger, the frustrations may be the reasons for blacks having more hypertension and at younger ages than whites. As a kind of "proof," they point to middle-class blacks who live outside the ghetto. These blacks have blood pressure readings similar to those of middle-class whites—significantly lower than blacks of lower economic levels living in such high-stress areas as Detroit during the riots of the sixties.

The role race plays is hardly clear. Japanese living in Japan eat a high-salt, low-fat diet. The rate of hypertension and stroke, especially cerebral hemorrhage, is high. As Japanese move to Hawaii and accommodate to a kind of halfway house between Japan and the United States, both hypertension and stroke rates moderate and there is a rise in heart disease. Once they move to the

United States, the pattern is exactly the same as for other Americans—more heart disease and stroke.

Hypertension and Treatment

Hypertension left untreated, then, can lead to any number of complications as well as what could be a final one—a stroke. Sustained high blood pressure is generally associated with two of the three types of strokes. Hardening of the arteries with narrowing or blockage of the arteries accounts for 65 percent of all strokes (Chapter III). It is linked to hypertension, too. Embolic occlusions (embolic blockage or embolism) which account for another 10 or so percent of all strokes, are not usually related to hypertension. The type of stroke that has been linked more directly to high blood pressure is the result of hemorrhage. Cerebral (brain) hemorrhages result in about 20 percent of the total number of strokes.

Approximate Frequency of Various Types of Stroke

Blockage of arteries to the brain (thrombosis)	**65%**
Traveling plugs obstructing arteries to the brain (embolism)	**10%**
Brain bleeding (cerebral hemorrhage)	**20%**
Miscellaneous	**5%**

The risk of stroke in hypertensive persons is five times the stroke risk in persons with normal blood pressure, according to some estimates. Studies such as the Framingham study bear the estimates out. It is in those strokes resulting from cerebral hemorrhaging that the relationship between sustained high blood pressure and stroke is most apparent and more easily explained.

Think of an electric percolator. When it is working properly, coffee bubbles cheerfully through the stem and against the top. If the control in the motor goes bad, the heat isn't regulated. Instead of bubbling, the coffee may start boiling so vigorously that it can explode the top off.

· Blood pressure is somewhat similar. The higher the blood pressure, the greater the stresses on arterial walls —tending first to weaken them and then precipitating rupture and hemorrhage. Hemorrhagic strokes happen because the rupturing of the cerebral blood vessel severely alters the pressure relationship within the brain. This leads to devastating mechanical disruption of the brain·substance, a kind of "blowing one's top" similar to the exploding coffee maker. About 10 percent of the victims of this kind of stroke die within 24 hours.

Treatment of sustained hypertension helps to prevent these strokes, and treatment is often a matter of dedication and belief on the part of the patient. The patient must be dedicated to the knowledge that high blood pressure can suddenly or insidiously end his life. The patient must believe that high blood pressure needs continuous treatment for the rest of his life. High blood pressure is expensive to treat, because medications can be expensive. But the cost is cheap in comparison to what a stroke may cost or the value of the life of the person himself. Then, too, cerebral hemorrhages usually strike during the years of high productivity and family responsibility, with about one in ten happening in young men of military age. So the dedication and belief in the treatment of sustained high blood pressure can bear its own rewards.

Chapter XII deals more specifically with treatment as a part of preventing stroke.

Experimental Hypertension

In the study of a disease, an important milestone in developing a treatment is the experimental production of the disease. By having an easily produced experimental model of high blood pressure, we can learn more about high blood pressure disease. These models have been produced in the following manner:

1. In 1934, Dr. H. Goldblatt showed that if the blood supply to the kidney of an experimental animal was reduced (by means of a clamp on the kidney artery) a progressive elevation of the blood pressure ensued. Many years later, after this epochal research effort, we have come to learn that this form of experimental hypertension is due to the release by the damaged kidney of a substance called *renin*. A great deal of enthusiastic and productive effort has gone into this type of experimental high blood pressure in order to determine its relationship to human counterparts.

2. Another method of inducing high blood pressure experimentally is by giving an animal gross excesses of salt. In the rat, this will occur in about a year if the animal has been drinking a salt solution of one part salt to 100 parts water. If hormones from the adrenal gland are given in addition to salt, less time is required to produce the hypertension.

3. Stimulating certain parts of the brain alert the areas concerned with the defense-alarm reaction. (The animal is aroused for flight or fright.) If these areas of the brain are stimulated for days to weeks, a moderate sustained hypertension results.

4. In the 1950s, Russian investigators using techniques of conditioning dogs (originally worked out by the great physiologist Pavlov) produced high blood pressure. If one interferes with self-protective mechanisms of the animal and frustrates it, high blood pressure can result. By the same token a change in conditioning can reduce or abolish the hypertension.

These are just some of the many ways high blood pressure has been produced experimentally. The use of different hormones in experimental high blood pressure would be another entire chapter. But experimental high blood pressure is just that. It has added to our basic knowledge about human hypertension and will continue to do so. Although it hasn't provided any easy answers yet, it has given us solid clues.

Experimental hypertension, although artificial, narrows or controls the variables that can affect blood pressure. We have learned that there is no single cause of hypertension. We have learned, too, how to modify the variables that affect high blood pressure with the goal of controlling human blood pressure.

In a larger sense, the world is a living laboratory. In it, we have peoples of different cultures with varying patterns of behavior and ways of life. Studies of different peoples provide us with interesting observations and clues regarding high blood pressure. During the last twenty-five years, a large number of cross-sectional surveys have been performed all over the world.

The subject of exercise—hard labor versus sedentary activity—and its relationship to high blood pressure has been a concern. Mayan Indians whose work loads are considerable and various Polynesian males of the Cook Islands atoll, Puka Puka, have relatively low blood pressure. On the other hand, sedentary clerks in Calcutta, German contemplative monks, and inactive elders of the Kenyan Samburu tribe all have low blood pressures. Exercise—or lack of it—doesn't seem to influence the blood pressures of the peoples referred to. High blood pressure can be found in peoples who are accustomed to vigorous and sedentary activity. For example, Jamaican hill farmers, Caribbean sugar-cane plantation workers, and Indians in the tea plantations of Assam all have relatively high blood pressure, and they do hard work. Sedentary professional people in other parts of India, Czechoslovak teachers and clerks have relatively high blood pressures. Thus, it seems evident that exercise patterns according to culture do not affect blood pressure levels. (See figure.)

Salt intake has long been suspected to have a relationship to high blood pressure level. As with exercise, some of the evidence is contradictory.

Buddhist farmers of Thailand eat relatively large amounts of salt, yet they have a uniformly low blood pressure. The salt intake of the workers on the sugar plantations of St. Kitts is about one-half that of the Thai farmer, yet the workers tend to have high blood pressure. The salt intake of coastal New Guinea natives is far higher than the "salt-deprived" inland natives—but both groups have relatively high blood pressure.

These studies seem to point to evidence that there may be other factors involved than how much salt a person uses. Dr. Lewis K. Dahl of Brookhaven National Laboratory in Upton, N.Y., has studied high blood pressure-salt relationships. He is a vigorous proponent of less salt in the diet as a result of his studies among five different populations: Americans, Alaskan Eskimos, Marshall Islanders, Japanese, and South African Bantus. As salt intake increased, so did high blood pressure. Alaskan Eskimos use little salt and have little high blood pressure, while northern Japanese have the highest salt intake and the most high blood pressure. Americans whose use of salt falls in between the two have more high blood pressure than Eskimos but less than the Japanese.

Dr. Dahl warns that these studies are just that—studies. Regardless of salt usage, about one in four persons does not have high blood pressure. Studies with rats are indicative, too. On a high-salt diet, two to five per cent of the rats develop "malignant" high blood pressure and die within a short time. One in four remains normal, with normal blood pressure. The other animals develop varying degrees of high blood pressure.

These studies support the Framingham study, which

found no close correlation between salt intake and blood pressure levels. Although the amount of salt taken in the diet may not *cause* high blood pressure, it can adversely affect high blood pressure once that condition is established—from whatever cause.

Genetics may play a role, so that developing methods to identify those persons prone to high blood pressure could aid prevention. But until these methods have been better developed and widely used, Dr. Dahl feels that we all would do well to cut down on salt intake.

Psychosocial stress is the result of the interaction of personality and environment, and it is held by many researchers to be a significant factor in high blood pressure development. Many population groups have been studied. In general, the blood pressure is lower where there is a stable culture, where group members are more secure in the roles assigned to them.

These observations are interesting, but none of them are definitive. They do show the difficulties physicians face. There is no one cause of high blood pressure. What all of us can do, though, is watch our weight, cut salt usage, avoid tension, and get our blood pressure checked regularly.

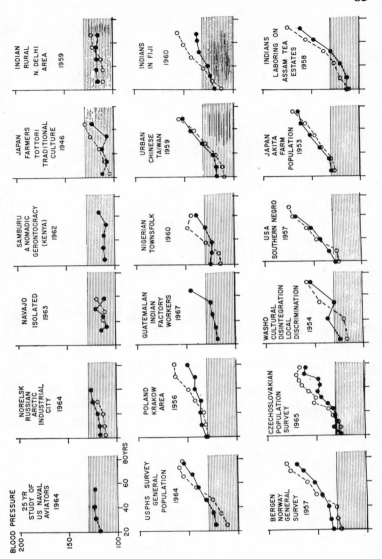

FIG. 4   BLOOD PRESSURE AND CULTURAL VARIA-
TION.   MALE—OPEN   CIRCLE;   FEMALE—
CLOSED CIRCLE.

From the *American Journal of Epidemiology* **90**, Nò. 3 (September 1969).
Reprinted by permission.

Chapter V

EMOTIONS AND EXERCISE

Is there a particular personality type who will have a stroke? Is the phlegmatic personality less likely to get a stroke than the enthusiastic personality? Does the extrovert run greater risks than the introvert?

The answer to all three questions is, "We don't think so."

At the same time, although there is no *one* well-defined personality type that gets stroke, just as there is no *one* physical type, it may be that the hard-driving, compulsive, ambitious person stands a better chance of having a heart attack or stroke—but this has been by no means proven as a result of studies. For example, the Minnesota Multiphasic Personality Inventory (MMPI) is composed of a series of tests designed to draw up personality profiles on the basis of questionnaires that bring out a person's responses to various life situations. Thus far, these tests have shown no direct relationship between types of personality and heart attacks or strokes. Perhaps future studies will reveal a specific personality stroke profile, but the point is that *anyone* and *everyone* can get heart attacks or have a stroke.

If mental disturbances, in and of themselves, were related to stroke, it would seem likely that we would find a higher incidence of stroke in mental hospitals. But mental disturbances and stroke don't seem to accompany each other. Mental hospitals, for example, have shown no disparity or close relationship between those patients with neuroses or psychoses and those with strokes. Even patients having electroshock therapy don't have more strokes than other patients. As a matter of fact, electroshock patients *rarely* get strokes, according to Dr. Lothar Kalinowsky.

Although we may rule out personality as a *direct* cause of stroke, we still cannot rule emotion entirely out as a contributing factor. Two points, however, have to be made clear:

1. Psychological factors *can* exert some effect on practically any illness, including high blood pressure and stroke.

2. A stroke or heart attack, by virtue of the illness and its consequences, may present the patient with a serious problem in psychological readjustment.

Louis Pasteur, whose "case history" was included in Chapter I, is one example of how both these points operate before and after a stroke. Within a very few years, his life pattern was upset by the death of his father and two daughters, all of whom he loved dearly. He had another emotional upset because of student riots at the university where he did his research and where he held an administrative position. Although he continued his research, he did lose his administrative job. Then there was his personality—hard-driving, compulsive, intense, somewhat humorless.

Since medical knowledge in his day was far inferior to what is available to us today, it is impossible at this time to gauge his physical condition. The fact remains that the internal pressures on him *may* have brought out an emotional response that could have contributed to his having his first stroke at the age of 44.

Emotions and Variations in Blood Pressure

Emotionally charged life situations may play a significant part in aggravating high blood pressure disease.

They do play some part in elevating blood pressure somewhat temporarily in normal people.

A group of medical students were studied just before a critical examination and then again a day or two later —after being informed they had passed. All the students were in general good health, with normal blood pressure readings, but just before the examination, their blood pressure rose. Afterwards, their blood pressure readings subsided to a normal level within a few days in practically all of the students. In this case, it can be safely assumed that tension or anxiety was responsible for the blood pressure elevations.

In contrast to this somewhat transient elevation under mild stress, more sustained hypertension has been observed when the stress has been of greater magnitude. Following the Texas City disaster in the midforties, 57 percent of the patients studied had blood pressures elevated above normal for as long as one to two *weeks* after the stressful situation. In another study, blood pressure readings were taken of a group of previously normal soldiers who were to be exposed to combat. Afterwards, 27 percent had developed high blood pressure, which was maintained in some of the men for as long as one to two *months* after they were out of combat and away from the source of the stress.

Disaster and combat are extremes of stressful situations. Equally emotion-loaded can be the drive along the freeway or expressway home from the office at night and to the office in the morning. Blaring horns, accidents, tie-ups in traffic, appointments to be met and kept, telephone calls, production schedules—these add stress in many forms. It may be excitement because of accidents avoided, tension to keep moving with the rest of the traffic, pressure because of the "prize" at the end of the drive. Also the "shelter" of the family may contain overt or hidden stresses.

There is also some evidence that some stressful situations are likely to be accompanied by significant elevations of serum cholesterol levels. Remove the stress and the levels drop, according to information gathered by Dr. Richard J. Jones at the University of Chicago School of Medicine.

Medical students, it seems, are not only a notoriously nervous lot but they also make good "guinea pigs." Medical students were studied before and after the day of final examinations. As anticipated, blood fat levels were lower when the exams were over. There are other scientists who are skeptical, however, and would like to see more extensive, controlled studies performed on the relationship of blood fats and the emotions.

Stress, then, is an unknown quantity. It is difficult to gauge. Not all people react to stress in the same way. Also, it is difficult to find out what the physical changes inside our bodies are. For this reason, a great deal of work has been done on animals.

A leading Canadian scientist, Dr. Hans Selye, spent a lifetime studying the effects of stress. Among many experiments he performed was one in which he took some healthy rats and conditioned them gradually with daily workouts on a treadmill, until he decided that they were physically fit through their heart rate and blood pressure readings. At this point, he subjected them to a wide variety of stresses. Horns blew, they were knocked about by blasts of compressed air and kept awake by flashing lights, electric shocks stimulated them. At the end of two weeks, they were as healthy as they were before the experiment.

Selye then took the same kind of rats and subjected them to the same stresses—with the exception that these rats were not conditioned. Before the end of the experimental two-week period, every single rat was dead.

There have been many other tests with animals. In another experiment, rats were subjected over a long period of time to forms of stress similar to those Selye used. All showed a rise in blood pressure, with changes in the kidneys and the adrenal glands that manufacture epinephrine (adrenalin), a substance secreted during stress. In another instance, cats were exposed to hostile dogs, with 50 percent of the cats showing elevated blood pressure as well as some kidney and heart damage.

The late Dr. Walter B. Cannon, a great physiologist, described the response of animals to flight or fright. Epinephrine poured into the circulation does increase blood pressure and increase the heart rate. Blood is also redistributed to allow for flight or fright. There is no question that stressful situations *can* cause elevated blood pressure in humans—but this is a far cry from saying that blood pressure disease is caused by stress alone. There are too many other causes of hypertension yet undefined.

Some people may have a vigorous emotional response, with consequent elevation of blood pressure, to a situation that may leave other people "cold." Phlegmatic types may respond with normal blood pressure readings. The "hyperreactors," whose blood pressure rises dramatically, have what is called *labile hypertension*. Lability correlates with anxiety—either overt or below the surface.

Blood pressure normally fluctuates—that is, it is lower during sleep or bed rest, higher during exercise or when one is under tension. If blood pressure rises to levels out of proportion to the stimulus, it is called labile hypertension. Some people—such as those who are clearly neurotic with severe anxiety—who would be thought to have labile hypertension have a normal blood pressure.

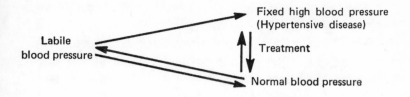

NORMAL VS. LABILE HYPERTENSION

Labile hypertension does not mean that a person's blood pressure only over-reacts a few times. It means a repeated, consistent reaction and is often accompanied by palpitation, irregular heartbeat, sweating, and tremor—the typical symptoms of anxiety. Although these symptoms may indicate other illnesses, e.g., over-activity of the adrenal and thyroid glands, they are most often due to anxiety. Although any person, man or woman, of any age may have labile hypertension, young people in their teens or twenties and women during menopause—both periods of high stress for those concerned—are frequent "victims." As a result, there have been attempts to "decondition" patients with labile hypertension through suggestion and reassurance. Results are too limited to draw any conclusions, and no one is sure whether the cause is all mental or may also be physical, perhaps even genetic. There is some solid evidence to suggest that high blood pressure does have some genetic base.

Not all hyperreactors have labile hypertension. The mechanism triggering reaction to overexcitement may not be thoroughly understood, but it is understood enough to know that such stress can trigger a heart attack or stroke. A perfect example is the excitement aroused in fans at sports events. Just about every sports arena, ballpark, stadium, or race track of any size has a physician or nurse on duty or available to treat emergencies, including the heart attack or stroke that may occur.

The "sudden death" overtime can have more specific meaning than that of a fight-to-the-finish sports event, and sports writers who write about "cardiac finishes" are using more than clever words.

Mr. D.B.A. is a 62-year-old sports fan who ate a hearty supper before attending the harness races on a hot, humid night in August. He had been advised to lose weight and to have his high blood pressure treated but ignored the advice, saying he would do both "soon." He placed a large bet on a favorite horse. He saw it enter the home stretch and didn't remember another thing until three days later, when he awakened from a coma. He had suffered a cerebral hemorrhage as the horses headed for home. The excitement elevated his blood pressure above what it already had been and caused bleeding within the brain. He took a year to recover fully. The stroke he had could have been prevented, and his horse had lost the race—he had lost all around.

Not only sporting events, but also other public or private events that are accompanied by intense emotional responses sometimes cause susceptible individuals to have strokes or heart attacks. Stress, or excitement, doesn't have to be associated with "fun" either.

Stress may play a role in hypertension among blacks living in ghetto areas, although the pressures of modern-day city life may reflect on anyone. Crime in the streets is more than a political issue in all large cities, and fear is as powerful an emotion as excitement. The elderly in particular may be susceptible to fear, knowing they are more vulnerable in being less able to protect themselves. All too often, older people are the victims of muggers for this very reason. An added handicap for older victims is that they are in the stroke-prone age to begin with, so the added stress may result in a serious cerebral accident.

Mrs. H.R. is a 70-year-old black woman who was in good health. She lived in New York City all her life but had been little bothered by the rise in street violence until she was mugged while taking a subway home from her daughter's house. The mugger threw her down the subway stairs. She was hospitalized, and X rays showed neither skull nor brain injuries. Three days later, she suffered a stroke. Fortunately, she recovered without disability.

Was the stroke brought on by "flight and fright?" We think so. We do know that such emotional stress can raise the blood pressure and that such elevations of blood pressure increase the risk of stroke. At the same time, there is still much to be learned about these relationships and how they work. There is also the suggested relationship of the Selye experiment, that good physical conditioning may enable us to respond with less danger to our blood pressure.

We might be healthier emotionally and have better blood pressure responses, then, if we can follow these basic "commandments":

1. If you have to make a decision, make it. Right or wrong, the decision has been reached and uncertainty is over. Prolonged indecision may create strong emotional stress.

2. We may be better off if we settle for "second place." Trying to be Number One *all the time*— in jobs, sports, and so on—involves stress that can make a winner a loser.

3. Being kind to others generally brings kindness in return. Kindness and consideration may be a condition for a long, happy life. We know that recovery from a stroke depends a lot on the

tender, loving care of family and friends. The same love and care applied in time may also contribute to preventing a stroke.

Exercise

The Selye experiment mentioned earlier suggested a relationship between being in good physical condition and the ability to offset the flight-and-fright mechanism. Physical condition suggests exercise.

"Sedentary should be spelled easy," according to Dr. Richard H. Waltier, medical consultant to the Physical Fitness Program of the YMCA of Greater New York. Occupation means little, he says. Mr. John Doe may be an unskilled laborer, a clerk, or a successful business-man.

"Daily he goes through his work habits; comes home to eat a heavy, fattening dinner," continues Dr. Waltier. Then he slumps into his favorite easy chair to watch Dr. Welby on TV. He stays in that chair munching creamy cakes or guzzling beer and presses the remote control buttons held in his hand to change the station to catch the Knicks. During half-time, he gets into his car and rides 3,000 feet to obtain a new supply of beer and a pack of cigarettes. He would have been much better off if he had walked or run the round trip and forgotten the purchases.

"Automation in business, construction, industry, professions, and in the simple functions of daily life has stultified and eliminated muscular activity from modern man." We are, in short, chair-borne *and* car-borne.

Would physical fitness in man enable him to resist the deleterious effects of flight-and-fright stress that Selye managed to do in rats by getting them in good physical shape? We can look to a few of the studies that have been made in man, although they are not controlled in the sense that one group of men took exercise while a second with similar work habits did not.

A study in Great Britain of middle-aged men found that death rates from coronary disease over a long-term period were higher among men whose work involved little physical activity (bus drivers and telephone operators) than among those whose work involved some movement (conductors and postmen). Studies in Israel have reported similar findings.

The invaluable Framingham Study has played a part in such studies, too. It used five indices to gauge activity and fitness: the total daily activity of work and leisure, lung capacity, heart rate, relative weight, and handgrip strength. Those persons adjudged to be fitter had fewer fatal heart attacks than the ones who were less fit. Light to moderate exercise, it seems, was beneficial.

With all this talk of exercise, what happens to us when we exercise?

Practically everyone has experienced the thumping in the chest, rapid pulse, red face, and profuse sweating that accompanies vigorous physical exercise. These changes are due to the increased force and rate of contraction (beat) of the heart, accompanied by an increase in blood pressure. The arteries of the muscles are dilated, bringing to the muscles the increased amounts of blood necessary for exercise. Once again, as in emotional reactions, the adrenal gland pours out hormones enabling us to respond with an increase in heart rate, blood pressure, and a redistribution of blood to our muscles.

Is it good to exercise this vigorously? Most experts feel that some exercise is important for physical as well as psychological reasons. If you are doing exercise that you enjoy and like to do, it will make you feel better and give you a positive mental outlook. The big proviso is that you are doing exercise consistent with your existing health and your interests. It isn't very rewarding to play golf if you can't stand the game, no matter how much good the exercise is for you.

It also isn't very rewarding to do strenuous exercise, if you have high blood pressure, are overweight, and smoke—because you might be exercised into the next world! If you go out and do some violent exercise without preparing for it with practice and training, you will be asking for trouble. So don't do violent exercise unless you are conditioned for it.

The typical example of what happens in this case is the normally sedentary man who goes out after a blizzard and shovels snow. Mr. J.G. is an office manager of a large computer firm. One morning in winter, he awakened to find the driveway drifted in with a heavy, wet snow. He got up, dressed, and had a heavy breakfast. Then he put on boots and an overcoat and went out. About an hour later, he had managed to clear away about a quarter of the drive. He was perspiring, his heart was beating quickly, his face was red with exertion. Instead of stopping and resting, he went on shoveling. A half hour later, he collapsed.

Luckily, his wife looked out the kitchen window and saw him. She called their physician, and Mr. J.G. was hospitalized. Fortunately, he survived—but hundreds of other men are not so lucky each winter. Unused to exercise, these men push themselves past their limits. Used to exercise, they might be able to survive the strain on their cardiovascular system.

The term "unused to exercise" brings up another school of thought about exercise based on the adage, "If you feel the urge to exercise, lie down until it passes." This school of thought suggests that the evidence that hardening of the arteries is prevented or reversed by exercise is inconclusive. It further claims that serious harm is done by abuse of exercise and consequently that exercise should be avoided entirely.

Moderation between strenuous and no exercise is probably the best policy.

Logically, people between 40 and 60 years of age should avoid exercises requiring great speed and strength. Those exercises that *train* endurance can be of value. Gymnastics, swimming, walking, golfing, bicycling, riding (horseback, that is, not cars), tennis doubles and so on can be interesting and healthy if done *regularly* and not just once in a while. In addition, there are bonuses. A pleasantly tired body can seduce even the most active mind into good sleep.

After the age of 60, more care should be used to avoid undue strain or stress. Walking, bicycling, and home exercises are of value. The Y's and other groups often offer regular programs, requiring physical examinations to be sure the program is consistent with the member's health and abilities.

Having a friend or friends join you for activities within your limits is a good method of doing regular, enjoyable exercising. But group activities aren't necessary. Doing sitting-up exercises in the confines of your dwelling can be just as rewarding and beneficial.

Here are three simple "commandments":

1. Exercise *regularly,* consistent with your age and interests and with your physician's advice and concurrence.
2. Condition yourself. Start lightly for a short period of time and build up your activities to the point of *pleasant* fatigue—do *not* exercise to the point of exhaustion.
3. *Enjoy* yourself in your exercise.

CHAPTER VI

STROKE AND ENVIRONMENT

A car's motor runs down because of rust that may clog the fuel lines and the various gases in the exhaust that erode the muffler. These are internal causes of aging, some of which can be prevented by tune-ups and maintenance, but there are also external influences aging the car. If you live in a northern state, salt compounds used during the winter to melt the ice on streets and roads affect the underside of the car. If you live at the seashore, prevailing winds off the ocean carry salt that corrodes or tarnishes the metal much faster than if you live inland.

A car, then, is subject to *interior* changes because of the type of gas and oil and even maintenance. It is also subject to exterior changes because of climate and weather—the environment. Little can be done about exterior influences, although the weight of oil can be changed for cold or hot weather and you can use antifreeze in the radiator to inhibit freezing.

Our bodies are subject to similar outside influences. High blood pressure and hardening of the arteries are related to the internal functions of the body and its organs—its physiology. Food is the body's fuel, and the arteries its life lines. The saying that you are what you eat needs modification. It should be: You are what you eat, what you think, what you do. If you eat right (low fat), think right (don't worry), do right (get regular exercise), you will be right—if your genetics are right.

Our health is a composite mixture of our genetics (our internal makeup) and environmental influences. The environmental factors are what we breathe, what we eat and drink, and all the pressures we have to react to.

The way our bodies maintain themselves, regardless of outside influences or climate, is owing to a mechanism known as homeostasis. This accounts for the internal order of things. The body, through its wisdom, has remarkable powers of regulating its internal processes. There are feedback, as well as compensatory, regulating phenomena that adjust to variations within and without the body.

The body's response to *external* factors constitutes the response to the environment. What we eat, drink, smoke, medicate, breathe, sense—all can affect body responses.

What effect does environment have on stroke? What does the type of water we drink, hard or soft, the altitude, whether we live in a hot or cold climate mean to us in terms of stroke possibility?

There are geographic patterns to stroke that, according to various studies, do not follow the pattern of heart disease. In the United States, stroke as a cause of death is more prevalent in the southeastern states, with the least number of strokes occurring in the southwestern and mountain states. The authors of the study making this finding, in trying to explain the geographic differences, examined death certificates for variations in diagnosing the cause of death as stroke. There weren't enough differences in the methods to account for the reason why stroke deaths were higher in one area than in another. One theory attempted to explain the geographic variations by diet, another by work patterns. Suffice it to say, we really don't know the reason for the difference or even whether the difference is real and not a statistical quirk.

These interesting statistics remain just that. They may be weighted artificially by virtue of a population move to the South and other, more subtle, factors, including the way physicians report causes of death.

The same argument of environment versus diet has been used to account for the high death rate from strokes in certain parts of Japan, where the rates were higher for the northeast and southwest areas. There, the geographic distribution of stroke coincided with the prevalence of high blood pressure, along with a diet composed mainly of rice and a high salt intake. In Japan, it is often assumed that a person died of cerebral hemorrhage without further substantiation.

Astrologists might be able to find a reason for the geographic differences because of the pull of the moon or the planets, but that answer won't satisfy the scientific spirit in us. Even so, coincidences, so far unexplainable, do seem to abound.

In Japan, as well as in the Scandinavian countries and England, the highest rates of stroke deaths have occurred in those areas where the temperatures were the lowest, according to studies investigating climate. If geography and climate do play some kind of role in stroke, it's possible for further research to find a link. One line of this continuing research concerns water.

Water and Stroke

Hard water is what causes the ring around the bathtub. It prevents soap and shampoo from making suds. It's the reason for all sorts of "softening" products to soften not only water but also the skin. Hard water, therefore, seems less desirable to many consumers.

Hard water does not mean that some water is "harder" than other water in the sense that one mattress is harder than another. Hard water is simply water with relatively high concentrations of calcium and magnesium, and the higher the concentration, the harder the water. At the same time, no water is probably absolutely soft—that is, completely free of calcium and magnesium, unless it is distilled water.

Anyone who has ever lived in a hard-water area, however, is very aware of the minerals, since they are deposited in the bottoms of tea kettles when water is boiled, with the deposits gradually building up so that it takes longer and longer to boil water. A steam iron is another gauge of hard water. Directions to many irons contain warnings to use distilled water—water with the minerals distilled or boiled out. Otherwise, mineral deposits clog the steam holes. Despite the effects hard water has on tea kettles and irons, the minerals in the water have nothing to do with the fitness of the water to drink in the sense of causing infection or spreading disease.

Although hard water has been a boon to advertising as a cause for all sorts of water-softening systems and products for over thirty years, it was only in 1957 that any relationship between the chemical nature of water and cerebrovascular disease was suspected in a Japanese study of stroke and geography. Since then, some relationship has been found to exist in other countries, including Great Britain and the United States.

Ironically it is soft—not hard—water that may be the ally of stroke. Soft water was linked to stroke in a study reported in England in 1973. In this study 245 men living in six separate English and Welsh towns with soft water low in calcium were compared with 244 men living in towns where the water was hard with a high level of calcium. All the men had lived at least twenty years in their particular areas. Leaving as little to chance as possible, the investigators checked the men for blood pressure, blood cholesterol levels, heart rate, and their smoking habits.

There were noticeable differences between the men

living in soft- and hard-water towns. In the soft-water towns, blood pressure, cholesterol, and heart rate were all higher. Since smoking patterns were similar, the differences between the groups was not in whether they smoked or how much. Their ages did seem to make some difference, however. The men between the ages of 40 and 50, regardless of group, tended to have similar blood pressure readings, cholesterol levels, and heart rates. But the men between 56 and 65 who lived in the soft-water towns had markedly higher levels than those in the hard-water towns.

Soft water, these investigators seemed to feel, may be related to the "sudden deaths" of stroke and heart attacks, as well as to sustained high blood pressure.

Other studies have also dealt with hard water versus soft water. London, for example, has hard water and Glasgow, Scotland, has soft water. Again, soft water seemed to be related to the higher rate of *sudden* death but not to the overall rate of deaths due to heart attacks.

England is no different than the United States. While "bigger" is not necessarily "better," a study in America involved an area with more than 7 million inhabitants who lived along the Ohio, Columbia, Missouri, and Colorado rivers. When it came to *non*cardiovascular deaths, all four river basins' mortality statistics were virtually the same, regardless of the hardness or softness of the water. Deaths due to high blood pressure and heart disease were another matter. The areas with hard water had consistently lower death rates than those with soft water. In all, 140 counties were involved, and they were selected not only because of the dissimilarity of their water but also because they were similar in population size and the size of their towns and villages.

A study in Sweden in 1965 found that people living in hard-water areas had lower rates of stroke than those living in soft-water areas. Investigators in Holland in 1967 found a similar link. These studies were all reported in "Geochemical Environment in Relation to Health and Disease," published in 1972 by the New York Academy of Sciences.

The ecology movement of the past few years has brought up the question of water pollution—"Is this water fit to drink?" A better question for stroke prevention may be, "Is this water *too* soft to drink?"

No one really knows for sure, and statistics tell only part of the story. There is a certain irony, however, in the fact that hard water has been considered less desirable because it leaves a scum in a bathtub and deposits that build up in steam irons and tea kettles. Yet hard water, for some unknown reason, may react within the body to leave fewer "deposits" than soft water. We just don't know enough about it yet. We need more studies on the effect hard and soft water have on atherosclerosis and high blood pressure.

Cadmium and Sustained High Blood Pressures

Calcium and magnesium in hard water aren't the only elements that may be related to stroke. Another is cadmium.

It used to be estimated that the value of all the minerals found naturally in the human body was about 99 cents. With inflation, that price has risen as spectacularly as other prices—but the point is that cadmium is one of the rare minerals found in the body. Somewhat similarly to the way inflation works the amount goes up as the person grows up. There even a geographic effect, again similar to inflation, which isn't the same for everyone in one country or in the world. A newborn baby has only a trace of cadmium present in its kidneys, but the amount increases, particularly in the first twenty years of life. Cadmium also accumulates in the liver, but it is the kidneys that seem to collect it. Because of the relationship of the kidneys to sustained high blood pressure, cadmium has come under some suspicion in relation to sustained high blood pressure. And, since sustained high blood pressure is also related to stroke, cadmium may play a role in both.

For one thing, sustained high blood pressure or hypertension varies from population to population and from one part of the world to another—and so does cadmium in the kidneys, depending on geography and environment. As an example, in areas in Africa where there is little hypertension, there is also a low level of cadmium in the kidneys. On the other hand, in areas of Japan where there is a high rate of hypertension, there is also a relatively large amount of cadmium in the kidneys.

The hypothesis that cadmium collects in the kidneys —the more the cadmium, the higher the rate of hypertension—has been tested in the laboratory. Rats have been given cadmium in their drinking water from birth until death. With time, they developed hypertension. That is, their blood pressure was significantly higher than that of rats who had not been given the cadmium-treated water. In addition, the cadmium-fed rats had shorter life spans. On the positive side, the cadmium-induced hypertension was *reversed* when the rats were fed medication that had the same effect on the rats as anti-hypertensive drugs have on humans.

Studies in man show that a newborn baby has almost no cadmium in its tissues and that cadmium accumulation increases with age. Part of the accumulation of this non-essential but potentially toxic metal may be due to diet. A Veterans' Administration Hospital study, however, traces some of the cadmium to cigarettes.

Cigarette tobacco contains cadmium, which is inhaled with the smoke. According to this study, the kidneys and liver of smokers contain more cadmium

than those of non-smokers. This would also help to
account for the reason why cadmium accumulation
seems to plateau in middle age and then decreases, since
smoking seems to be heaviest between the ages of 25
and 40. After that, smoking habits change, with many
smokers either cutting consumption or giving up cigarettes entirely.

Again, as with hard water, there is still much to be
learned about where the cadmium comes from and why,
and how it affects the kidneys the way it does. Until
such time, judgment has to be reserved on the relationship between stroke, high blood pressure, and cadmium.

The Total Environment and Stroke

The effect of the total environment on persons is difficult to gauge. Most people live in the same or similar
environments all their lives. If they move, perhaps one
factor in the environment will be changed—such as
moving from a hard- to a soft-water location, or from a
cold or temperate climate to a hot or tropical one, as
when people retire to Florida or the Southwest. But
most factors will be relatively unchanged. People who
live and work in a city will move or transfer to another
city, for example.

What would happen, however, if the total environment were drastically changed, if a group of people
were to move from one location to a completely different one, socially and economically and geographi-
cally at variance with the original one? This is what
happened when the Yemenites moved to Israel.

Yemen is a small, mountainous country on the southwestern tip of the Saudi Arabian peninsula in the Middle East. Economically, it could be called "underdeveloped." Until 1949, Yemen had a fairly sizable Jew-
ish population that then emigrated to the newly formed
state of Israel. The Yemenites, who are considered Oriental, were a serene group with a devout belief in their

religion. They left Yemen on foot, traveled long distances under incredible hardships, until they arrived at embarkation points where they were ferried by airplane to Israel. So primitive had been their living conditions in Yemen that, to them, the airplane was a kind of Biblical miracle transporting them by magic carpet to the Promised Land. Most of them had not only never seen an airplane; they had also never benefited from electricity or modern plumbing.

The dominant figure in the Yemenite family is the male, whose authority has been unquestioned and unchallenged. According to purely Yemenite custom, he was permitted more than one wife. The process of assimilation is a slow one, however. Yemenite villages have been created in Israel. There, the Yemenites' mode of behavior and social customs are being perpetuated. Their chief occupations are skilled production of handicrafts and raising poultry.

In the 1950s, heart attacks were rare in all Oriental Jews, who include the Yemenites, Jews from North Africa, Syria, Iraq, and other eastern countries, who comprise 25 percent of the total Israeli population. There were, in fact, only 2 cases of Yemenites having heart attacks out of a total of 412 heart attacks investigated in one study. When the cholesterol levels of the Yemenites were investigated over a twenty-year period, it was noted that the cholesterol levels rose from a low of approximately 160 milligrams to more than 200 milligrams. North African Jews and people from the Atlas Mountains in Morocco also had low blood cholesterol levels and a correspondingly low incidence of heart attacks. Those originating from the Atlas Mountains, however, have high blood pressure readings, which may be related to their high consumption of salt. Among the many excellent studies performed and work done in these areas was that of Professors Fritz Dreyfuss and Otto Streifler.

Interestingly enough, as far as environment is concerned, as these Jews assimilate, there is an increased incidence of stroke, especially among those from North Africa. An Israeli study examined hardening of the arteries of the brain among Jews of European and of Afro-Asian origins. The degree of hardening of the arteries of the brain was similar in both groups, but twice as many Afro-Asians (25 percent) showed evidence of stroke and stroke symptoms (transient ischemic attacks) as did Europeans (12 percent). What is more, when it came to heart attacks, the opposite ratio seemed true, with 40 percent of those Europeans, and only 15 percent of the Afro-Asians examined showing evidence of either an acute or old heart attack. Sustained high blood pressure was not a factor—16 percent of both groups had histories of high blood pressure, regardless of whether the cause of death was stroke or heart attack.

What are the reasons for the difference? A possible explanation may be that those members of the European group who might develop hardening of the arteries of the brain severe enough to kill them have heart attacks before this can happen. By the same token, the Afro-Asians' risk of dying from stroke may be increased because they do not run as high a risk as the Europeans of dying from heart disease before the stroke occurs. Because of the difference between the two groups, environment may be a factor. The changed environment of the Yemenites has resulted in changes of their cholesterol levels, for one thing.

The influence of diet as a part of the total environment comes out in the Yemenites in another way. In the twenty years since their arrival in Israel, they averaged a 20-pound weight gain and had an increased incidence of diabetes. Although their diets in Yemen included little sugar, that changed in their new environment.

Cigarette smoking has not been considered a factor either for or against the rising incidence of stroke and heart disease. The Yemenites continue to use water pipes for smoking, and the water apparently acts as a shield protecting them from the ravages of tobacco.

We may conclude, then, that as the Yemenites have adapted to their new environment, there were physiological changes, with an increase in heart disease and stroke, perhaps due to changes in diet, perhaps because of social changes and resulting psychological changes in moving from an underdeveloped to a highly developed country. One theory is that the Yemenite male is having an identity crisis now that more than one wife is being frowned upon.

The simple fact is that no one knows for sure how important environment may be. If it does have a bearing on stroke, we still have much to learn about which of the many factors may be more important than the others.

Other Factors

Aside from the natural minerals found in water, there are additives. Most drinking water in America, Great Britain, and other Western countries is treated in some way to purify it. The most common water purifying agent is chlorine, a heavy, greenish-yellow gas that is used in many sterilizing methods.

Although the minute quantities of chlorine in tap water and in flour are considered safe, chlorine does have a smell and a taste in larger quantities—as anyone who has swallowed water in a swimming pool can testify. Even though the amount used in a pool is more than what comes out of the tap, it isn't enough to make a person ill. The purpose of the stronger concentration in the pool is to avoid the danger of infection or disease being passed through the water.

Regardless of the proven safety of chlorine since it was first introduced to purify water in 1875, every once in a while someone complains about the supposed effect of chlorine on people. Some relate the chlorination of water over the past century to the rise in hardening of the arteries. There are claims made that it causes fat to deposit in the rubber and metal tubes of milking machines as well as in artificial vein and artery grafts and the human circulation system—the familiar plaques of hardening of the arteries. Links are made between highly chlorinated water and the high incidence of hardening of the arteries in the American soldiers who were killed in action and autopsied during the Korean and Vietnam wars. All drinking water, therefore, according to proponents of this theory, should be boiled since boiling sterilizes and removes the chlorine. In addition to boiling water, advocates of this theory propose a diet composed of milk, cheese, eggs, meat, poultry, fish, and butter—foods that contain large amounts of cholesterol and saturated fats, which others feel are involved with hardening of the arteries.

Although it is true that hardening of the arteries and stroke have increased during the past century, particularly in affluent Western society, there may be other reasons for the increase. For one thing, medical science (through the control of disease, better sanitation, and the providing of better medical care) has lengthened the life span tremendously. The effects of hardening of the arteries do not become apparent, in general, until a person reaches the 50s, and more people are living to this age and older. Thus, there would be an increase in the diseases of aging as the life span lengthens. We think one reason for a low rate of these diseases in countries without chlorinated water and bleached flour may be that the people don't live long enough to develop them.

We do know that chlorinated water can prevent disease. Whenever chlorination is omitted or is not adequate there seems to be an outbreak of disease. Even deep wells, usually thought to be safe, may become tainted. This was the case in an outbreak of Salmonellosis, a severe kind of "stomach flu" normally linked to tainted food, in a California town in 1965. Somehow harmful bacteria got into the water system. Chlorination ended the outbreak. More recently in 1973, at the height of the tourist season in Miami Beach, there was a scare of typhoid. An outbreak of typhoid at a farm labor camp in Homestead, near Miami, was directly linked to the breakdown of a chlorinating unit.

The relationship of chlorine to hardening of the arteries is possible but unlikely. Until there is positive proof, chlorination of drinking water is probably the safest, as well as the most economical, way to purify water.

In short, then, we simply do not know enough yet to be sure what factors in our environment are related to hardening of the arteries, sustained high blood pressure, heart disease, and stroke—and in what way. Environment may be like genetics: If we could pick our "druthers" of where to be born, grow up, and live, we should pick a place where there is a low rate of death from stroke, with hard water containing nearly no cadmium, in the southwest or one of the mountain states, where the climate is not too cold. Such a place would be ideal, a veritable Garden of Eden without the snake of stroke to spoil it. But there is still too much to be learned about the effects of environment before we decide where Eden is.

In any disease process, such as hardening of the arteries or sustained high blood pressure, the exact causes of which are unknown, the public must be protected against misleading statements, curealls, and magic nostrums. There are always and will always be fringe groups who are interested in promoting a particular point of view because of mistaken conclusions or worse. Even so, we must encourage differences of opinion among our scientific community in order to abet the spirit of inquiry and observation that is vital to progress.

Chapter VII

"MEDICINE-SHOW MEDICINE" AND STROKE

The "medicine show" was once a standard part of our American culture. It was also, in many ways, the ancestor of American advertising, in that it offered entertainment leading up to a hard-selling pitch for some kind of nostrum or panacea. For 50 cents or a dollar a bottle, the purchasers were offered a head-to-toe cure for everything from dandruff to flat feet—and all the ailments of the body in between. The pitchmen had their spiel down pat, and they knew how to trade on the audience's desires and human susceptibility with promises of a magic or secret cure.

The medicine shows are gone, and we have the Federal Drug Administration to keep an eye on "magic potions." But the pitchmen are still with us, and so is the all too human susceptibility to their promises.

The hard facts are that heart disease and stroke can't be cured by magic. They may be prevented and the underlying causes treated—but only through the help of modern medicine. Although medical scientists are searching for a cure for hardening of the arteries and high blood pressure, we have so far found only methods of treating the implications of these diseases.

We know that diet can have an effect on both diseases, elevating blood fats and aggravating hardening of the arteries and raising blood pressure. We know that diet may also arrest or even reverse them. The best diet thus far devised is probably the prudent diet.

We know, too, that cigarettes have an effect on blood pressure and hardening of the arteries. Yet, led by clever advertising techniques, backed by powerful economic interests, the health of millions now goes up in smoke every year.

The claims of a "safer" cigarette and a "magic" diet are as attractive today as the claims of medicine-show pitchmen used to be. They are a kind of wild pitch, with the claims as wild as what is often being "pitched."

Alcohol has had a similar history. Originally thought of as an elixir of life, it has become an abused drug, one that can ruin lives and even kill if the desire to overindulge takes over.

Of all three—diets, cigarettes, and alcohol—diets are probably the most popular staple of the medicine show. Every year a different diet is touted either for "health" reasons or to "lose" weight. Many of them do not take into account the basic elements of nutrition, while others are based on a momentary trend. Still others are bizarre, making outrageous claims for impossible cures on the basis of eliminating certain foods and adding others. There is a world of difference between those diets and a low-cholesterol, prudent diet, a low-salt diet for high blood pressure, or a special diet for diabetes.

A *prudent diet* makes no claims that it can completely prevent hardening of the arteries, since this is a normal process of the body, although the advance may be reversed in some cases. Again, although a low-cholesterol diet avoids certain foods, it includes all the nutrients we need.

A *prudent diet* is medically approved.

Food Faddism

Much of food faddism is based on misinformation and wish fulfillment as far as health is concerned. Although not all of this food faddism is directly related to stroke, it is related to general good health. For this reason then, we should beware of any diet that makes outrageous claims for stroke, hardening of the arteries, high blood pressure, or any other disease. These fad diets are like a medicine-show shell game in which the consumer can't win. There are no miracle foods or diets.

Food faddism is often followed blindly, either against a doctor's advice or in preference to seeking competent medical advice. The follower may even put off seeing a physician when early care could save expensive treatment and even a person's life.

Fad diets fall into three types: fads in which a particular food is supposed to have curative powers for a specific disease; those in which the elimination of certain foods is supposed to enhance good health because eliminating the foods also eliminates harmful substances; and fads that emphasize "natural" or "health" foods at the cost of other foods.

One of the most persistent of the fad diets over the years has been the vegetarian diet. Although it crops up in many different forms in keeping with the times, a vegetarian diet falls into one of three categories:

1. Vegans, in which the followers don't eat meat, fowl, eggs, milk products, or fish.
2. Lacto-vegetarian, which denies its followers meat and fish but allows them to drink milk and eat butter and cheese.
3. Lacto-ovo-vegetarian, which permits drinking milk and eating eggs.

What may happen to you on these diets?

Nutritional deficiency is not likely to occur in either of the last two diets, because cow's milk does contain the essential amino acids and vitamin B-12 that the body needs. The vegans diet, however, lacks these essential amino acids.

The body itself manufactures certain amino acids it needs—but it cannot make all of them. Amino acids are the building blocks of protein. Protein is a combination of amino acids linked to one another. To make protein, the body needs both the amino acids it manufactures and those in foods. The amino acids in food that the body can't manufacture are called the "essential" amino acids, and they include isoleucine, leucine, lysine, phenylalanine, methionine, threonine, tryptophan, and valine. Infants require also histidine. Meat, fowl, fish, eggs, or milk are the only sources of *all* of these essential amino acids.

Any vegetable lacks one or more essential amino acid. For example, cereals are deficient in lysine; corn has a low tryptophan content; soybeans and seed oils are low in methionine; legumes (peas, beans, lentils) are low in methionine and tryptophan; peanuts lack methionine and lysine. Some mixtures of vegetables may probably provide all of the essential amino acids, but diets limited to only a few vegetable sources are likely to be deficient in some essential amino acids. In light of our present knowledge of nutrition, therefore, it is advisable that a vegetarian include skim milk or skim-milk cheese in his diet.

Even more harmful than a purely vegetarian diet is the Zen-Macrobiotic diet that in the past few years has found quite a few followers. It is an extreme example of what can happen on a fad diet. It has been associated with Zen Buddhism, although wrongly, and its followers believe that by adhering to it they can achieve spiritual rebirth (*Zen* means "medication," with *macrobiotic* meaning "longevity"). The diet is also supposed to cure diseases that run the gamut from dandruff to heart disease, making it a panacea or cure-all. Instead, serious nutritional deficiencies and some deaths have resulted among people on this diet, with anemia, scurvy (vitamin C deficiency), and low serum protein being reported.

Fluids, sugars, and meats are avoided completely. Fruits and vegetables are gradually eliminated until whole-grain cereals compose 100 percent of the diet. Reportedly the diet is now being rewritten to include sound nutritional principles. In the meantime, those who follow the diet strictly are asking for trouble.

A diet supplement for which the claims are just about as much as for the Zen diet is vitamin E. Despite studies showing that vitamin E in large doses has little or no effect, there are periodic claims dating from 1946 that it can benefit heart disease, including hardening of the arteries. Controlled studies have proven otherwise, but there are still claims that vitamin E can do just about anything that the old carnival snake oil could do, in curing every disease from A to Z. Vitamin E is the vitamin in search of a disease. Its use can hurt nothing except your pocketbook.

A diet that periodically turns up is the white rice diet. White rice is not a whole grain, as is the brown rice called for in the Zen diet. Although it does contain some *incomplete* proteins, proteins lacking essential amino acids, it contains no vitamins at all.

The results of a completely vegetarian diet can be found in some poor lands where there is a lack of protein, and the protein-deprived children suffer from serious physical and mental retardation. The only preventative is a diet including those essential amino acids found in meat and dairy products, but in these countries people are forced to rely on vegetable protein. They cannot afford these foods. Scientists are trying to develop new strains of legumes that will contain the essential amino acids. They are also seeking substitute foods. In Peru, a high-protein cereal found little acceptance, regardless of how healthful it was—it smelled and tasted like a wet dog. In Indonesia, a weaning drink for babies failed with children, but it became popular with the elite as a party drink.

Acceptance of foodstuffs is culturally oriented. In addition, the food must taste good. Nevertheless, America may be exceptional, since fad diets gain some acceptance, regardless of what the foods in them are.

Another form of food faddism concerns what have been called health, organic, or natural foods. It has received additional impetus in recent years because of a distortion in the ecology movement. There is little difference among the three.

A health food has certain benefits ascribed to it, perhaps on the basis of misinformation about vitamins that supposedly furnish energy or are supposed to help a particular condition, such as arthritis, a long-time favorite of food faddists. Organic, or organically grown, or natural foods are considered to be those grown without the use of any chemicals or processed without chemicals, or both. What is forgotten by advocates of these foods is that all foods are healthy, if the diet is a properly balanced one.

Chemical fertilizers and pesticides, which are the basis for the argument against commercially grown foods, have no proven effect on the food itself. All they do is increase the yield per acre. In addition, there is no proof that food grown with natural fertilizers is superior to commercially grown foods in taste or quality, according to many consumer guidelines. The nutrients within food are the same regardless of the way in which it is grown. Using natural (or organic) fertilizers may even be hazardous, since organic fertilizers are carriers of salmonella, a bacteria that manufactures a potent toxin responsible for food poisoning. Pesticides are regulated by law and within certain levels have been determined to be safe. "Organic foods" have a disadvantage in a time of high prices, too—they cost from 30 to 100 percent more than nonorganic groceries.

Natural foods are similar in many respects to health foods. Their producers disclaim the use of "artificial" additives, such as vitamins. Many claims may be false. In one instance, rose hips vitamin C tablets were found to be fortified with synthetic ascorbic acid (vitamin C); in another, natural vitamin B tablets had synthetic chemicals added.

A current demand for certified unpasteurized (raw) milk is a further example. Certified milk, produced in accordance with standards established by the American Association of Medical Milk Commissions, Inc., includes raw, pasteurized, homogenized, or milk fortified with vitamin D. Raw certified milk is expensive and it is also an excellent medium for growing bacteria so that, despite the standards, it may contain dangerous organisms. On the other hand, pasteurized milk is perfectly safe because of the high quality of the pasteurization equipment and controls.

Our present craze for vitamins may be carrying enough of a good thing too far. Dr. Charles Butterworth, Jr., director of the Nutrition Program at the University of Alabama School of Medicine, questioned fortifying milk with vitamin D. He said. "There is no evidence that adults require more vitamin D than the amounts naturally present in ordinary foods, and synthesized by the skin upon exposure to sunlight."

He added, "On the other hand, very large doses can cause hypercholesterolemia and coronary artery lesions in experimental animals. It remains to be seen if vitamin D is in any way related to the high incidence of atherosclerotic disease in this country, but the mere classification of a chemical compound as a vitamin does not guarantee its safety for prolonged use at unphysiological levels."

Cigarettes and Stroke

High blood cholesterol levels and elevated blood pressure have been proven to have a relationship to heart disease and stroke. The relationship of cigarettes to stroke is no less direct than it is to heart disease. Smoking is linked to so many diseases, both stroke-related and non-stroke-related, that it has to be considered a strong risk.

There is no one substance in cigarettes that can be isolated and given *all* the blame for either cancer or cardiovascular disease. When a cigarette burns, it produces a mixture of particles and gases. This mixture, all together, can irritate every part of the body's respiratory system and affect the cardiovascular system. The gases include not only a number of chemicals that, so far, have been found to be harmless but also such harmful ones as carbon monoxide, a lethal poison. The particles include tars that are irritating and are linked to cancer; nicotine, a potent drug; and small amounts of arsenic, an elemental poison.

As a person inhales, these poisons are absorbed into the body. What, then, if a person does not inhale?

Even though 90 percent of the nicotine is absorbed into the body by inhaling, up to 10 percent is absorbed by merely puffing a cigarette. Not inhaling, then, may be an answer to *reducing* the risk of heart disease and stroke, but it's not a solution. Pipe and cigar smokers, who don't inhale, do run less risk of cardiovascular disease. Yet their chances of *mouth cancer* may be slightly increased.

Smoking filter cigarettes for protection is a myth. Some filters do reduce the amount of nicotine, gases, and tars, but since the tars and nicotine are the very elements that make smoking "satisfactory," it would be impossible to reduce all of them. The result is, too, that as cigarettes become less satisfactory due to filters, smokers will often smoke more of them to get that satisfaction. Nevertheless, if they do *not* smoke more, if they smoke the *same* number of cigarettes or cut down, they may cut their chances of getting lung cancer. Still, the death rate for filter-tip smokers is higher than for people who do not smoke at all. There is no such thing as a safe cigarette at present. A lot of money is spent trying to find one.

Statistics gathered by the American Cancer Society show that men whose cigarette habit is less than a pack a day have a 60 percent higher death rate than nonsmokers; those whose habit is one to two packs a day, about 90 percent higher; and those whose habit is two or more packs a day, about 120 percent above nonsmokers. What's more, one-pack-a-day smokers of 25 years of age may be losing five and a half years of their lives in comparison to nonsmokers. At every age, it seems, cigarette smokers have a higher mortality rate than do nonsmokers, with 300,000 smokers dying unnecessarily each year from a number of different causes related to smoking.

Although most statistics pertain to men, the same factors are operating in women who, in general, have been smoking less, for shorter times, than men. On the other hand, the death rate of women smokers has been climbing so that it now parallels that of men, with a correspondingly increased risk of lung cancer and cardiovascular disease, including stroke. Women smokers who become pregnant also have a greater chance of stillbirths and have smaller babies, whose five and a half pound average weight (considered premature) makes the babies more susceptible to deaths in their first month of life.

The Surgeon General's report damned cigarette smoking in the midsixties. Tobacco sales did decrease for a few years, but then rose again, showing that millions of Americans not only smoke but are "enslaved" by a bad habit. The habit costs one-pack-a-day smokers at least $150 a year and two-pack-a-day smokers, at least $300, with the amount increasing each year because of new taxes and rising prices.

The cost of smoking is high—high in money and in health. Every study is consistent in showing how cigarette smoking affects cardiovascular disease.

What happens to you when you light a cigarette? The heart beats faster, blood pressure is raised, and the blood vessels of the skin, especially in the extremities, are narrowed and constricted. As long as a person is healthy, these changes are temporary, varying according to the person's reaction to tobacco. If the person already has any one of several diseases of the blood vessels (including hardening of the arteries), the condition can be aggravated by the increased constriction of already narrowed and damaged blood vessels.

The International Atherosclerosis Project and other international projects have confirmed that hardening of the arteries advances more rapidly if the person has sustained high blood pressure and/or diabetes—and if he smokes cigarettes. Autopsies are further proof that hardening of the arteries is more severe in the aorta and coronary arteries of those persons who were smokers than in those who had never smoked. If even more proof is needed, experiments with animals also show the influence of smoking, especially when the animals are fed a high-cholesterol diet.

These experiments involved dividing the test animals in two groups, both of which were fed a high-cholesterol diet. The one group was exposed to carbon monoxide levels of the amount that would be inhaled by habitual smokers. The other group was not exposed to any carbon monoxide. Although both groups had lesions due to hardening of the arteries, those in the animals that had breathed the carbon monoxide mixture were of greater extent and severity.

Another study, of which the Framingham study was one part, came up with more vital statistics at the human level. It dealt with the risk factors in cardiovascular disease individually and what happened when one risk factor was combined with another or with several factors.

The participants were asked whether they had ever smoked or if they had smoked in the past only. If they smoked, they were separated into those who were currently smoking pipes or cigars only and those who smoked less than half a pack of cigarettes a day, a package of cigarettes a day, and more than one pack a day. Of the group of those who had never smoked, fewer had major coronary "events" (less than 50 per 1,000 men over ten years) and deaths. Those who had smoked in the past and now smoked a pipe or cigars had 50 major events per 1,000 men over the ten-year period studied. The men who smoked less than half a pack of cigarettes a day had slightly more than 50 events per 1,000 men, with the rate rising rapidly to more than 175 events per 1,000 among those men who smoked more than one package a day.

When all three risk factors (cholesterol levels, blood pressure levels, and smoking) were combined, the results were even more startling. The men who had low cholesterol, normal blood pressure, and had never smoked had about 25 major coronary events per 1,000 and even fewer deaths from all coronary heart disease. If one of the three factors were involved, both rates almost doubled. If two risk factors were involved, the rate of major coronary events rose to slightly less than 100 per 1,000 men, with the number of deaths about 50. All three factors combined zipped the number of first major coronary events upwards to 175, with deaths rising to 75 per 1,000 men.

Cigarette smoking is a definite risk factor, then. Moreover, the younger in age the smoker is, the greater the relative risk.

Although all of these studies deal with coronary heart disease, a similar risk is involved in stroke. Atherosclerosis is not confined to the aorta or the coronary arteries, although it does start in the aorta at an early age. Cigarette smoking could be said to add insult to injury in the way it increases the advances of hardening of the arteries.

What happens when men change their diet habits, lower their blood pressure, and stop smoking? Atherosclerosis can be slowed down and even reversed to a certain extent. And this is what happened to the men in the Pooling Project.

Why cigarettes hasten hardening of the arteries, especially if the smoker eats a high-cholesterol diet, is under study. The exact mechanism is yet to be discovered. From other studies on the effects of cigarettes and general health, however, scientists have been able to isolate at least some of the substances in cigarettes that are harmful to health (nicotine, tars, and gases). Some of these have already been linked to cancer, especially cancer of the lungs, mouth, larynx, esophagus, and bladder.

Stopping smoking does help, and it's never too late to stop.

Many American physicians have given up smoking, although statistics on how many are not available. All anyone has to do for proof, however, is to attend a medical meeting. Whereas medical meetings were formerly attended by a great many doctors and a lot of smoke, the atmosphere has cleared to the extent that— while there is still fire at the meetings—there is hardly any smoke. Although physicians may not always follow their own advice, this is one instance where we are really practicing what we preach.

Why, then, do so many millions of Americans smoke, despite the fact that 29 million *have* quit smoking, according to Cancer Society statistics? These figures prove that people can stop smoking.

One reason is probably the advertising that abounds in magazines and newspapers, even if it is off television, making smoking seem desirable for any number of reasons, including sex. Another is that smoking is acceptable. Although airlines and other modes of public transportation have increased their bans on no smoking, the efforts of some people to prohibit people from smoking at all on planes or trains have met a strong wall of resistance. With smoking cars and smoking areas readily available, people smoke—sometimes for no other reason than that the person next to them does.

As far as young people are concerned, they tend to copy their elders, even though the elders may secretly wish they could stop smoking. The fact is that the younger a person is when he *or* she starts to smoke, the greater are the chances of lung disease or heart attacks or strokes before the 30s, or the 40s.

Alcohol and Stroke

Alcohol has been used since the dawn of history to dim the realities of the present. Alchemists in their unsuccessful quest to convert base metal to gold sought and felt they found a panacea and an elixir of life in alcohol. Actually, alcoholic beverages are not a panacea. Alcohol is a drug with some remarkable qualities, but like any other drug it has some bad side effects and may cause addiction, if abused.

Alcohol has had a varying history depending on social customs and environment. The ancient Hebrews used alcohol ceremonially and through experience found, that used externally, it sterilized, cooled, and disinfected the skin.

Interestingly enough, the true believers of Mohammed shun alcohol in any form: yet it was they who introduced the art of distilling into Europe in the Middle Ages. The use of wine and other spirits in all of Europe as a table beverage has had a long history, too. In Gaelic, whiskey means the "water of life." Aqua Vit, which is drunk throughout Scandinavia, also means "water of life" and was once used purely medicinally.

Regardless of its history in medicine, alcohol doesn't prevent strokes—nor does it cause them.

The chief benefit of alcohol in relatively small doses is its ability to blunt anxiety. It works by depressing the brain centers responsible for our inhibitions. If our inhibitions are blocked, we feel stimulated, which is why the misconception has grown up that alcohol is a stimulant. It isn't—it is a *depressant,* although by depressing inhibitions it may often give a sense of well-being and confidence to one who didn't feel that way before.

There are a certain number of physical changes, too. After a moderate drink of alcohol, there is a feeling of warmth accompanied by a reddening of the face, often flushing, because of the dilation of the arteries of the skin. There is no good evidence, however, that alcohol can increase the flow of the blood to the heart or the brain. Making you feel better may make alcohol in moderation a form of good medicine, though.

It may also help the digestion and appetite in the elderly, as well as relax them. If stress is a significant factor in stroke—which is still unproven but likely—alcohol may relieve the stress and by relieving the tension reduce the danger of stroke.

On the other hand, since alcohol is a drug and a medicine, like any other medicine it shouldn't be abused or taken if you have certain illnesses. Most physicians feel it can aggravate gastrointestinal ulcerations and also feel it definitely shouldn't be used by people with liver trouble. Persons with elevated fat levels in their blood may also be encouraged to limit alcohol intake. One recommendation restricts these patients to no more than two servings of alcohol a day, with the serving defined as:

> 1 ounce (a shot) of such alcohol as whiskey, vodka, gin, or rum
> 5 ounces of beer
> 2½ ounces of dry table wine
> 1½ ounces of sweet dessert wine, such as port or madeira

Despite the adage that "there are more old drunks than old doctors," abstainers or moderate drinkers live longer than heavy drinkers. On this basis, here are "three commandments" for drinking alcoholic beverages:

1. If you are used to drinking occasionally and it relieves you without adverse effects continue to drink moderately.
2. If you have a weight problem, remember that a quart of beer has about 500 calories; an ounce of whiskey, about 150 calories; and one wineglass has at least 120 to 150 calories.
3. If you can't stop drinking, don't start.

To sum up: What Shakespeare said is probably true: Alcohol "provokes the desire, but it takes away the performance," especially while driving! Whatever you have to do—for work or pleasure—you'll do better without the help of alcohol.

Chapter VIII

THE ANATOMY OF A STROKE

Have you ever tried to make a telephone call, only to find your phone was out of order so that you couldn't use it—or that your phone was working but the number you were calling was out of order? It's possible that the central switchboard was out of order in both instances.

A human brain is more complex than the most complex telephone switchboard; yet it does have a certain similarity. If the switchboard is partially out of order, incoming or outgoing calls can be affected—similarly with the brain. Incoming nerve impulses to the damaged brain are poorly received or not received at all, so that outgoing impulses may not be transmitted.

A switchboard also has to have a power source in order for electrical impulses—messages—to be sent. If the source breaks down, the finest switchboard in the world is useless, because power has failed. If the switchboard breaks down completely, the power will be useless.

Both examples are similar to what happens in the body. The heart is the pump providing supplies to the brain through the blood containing oxygen and glucose. Pump failure (heart attack) or plugs in the arteries to the brain can decrease supplies to the brain and this can decrease the source of power to the brain. The brain, our switchboard, weighs 3 pounds and receives 20 percent of the blood pumped by the heart per minute.

This brain-switchboard sends messages and instructions that enabled a printer to set the type on this page. The messages enable all of us to put one foot in front of the other, to move the fork unerringly from our plates to our mouths, to dress ourselves, all without thinking much about our actions. The difference between our brains and a switchboard is that the brain is also capable of wild flights of imagination and Einstein-like mathematical equations, independent of the need to move the body. The brain receives and integrates information and then transmits instructions for effective responses. A brain didn't write Shakespeare's plays—a hand did, responding to the brain.

When this brain-switchboard is partially damaged because of a switchboard failure, this may be analogous to an artery to a part of the brain being blocked because of a thrombus (plug) or an embolus (a traveling clot). A rupture of an artery or a blowout of an aneurysm does the same thing. And this is what happens to a brain in a stroke.

Just as a failure in a telephone switchboard is going to have an effect, either limited or extensive, on one or a few phones or all the phones in an area, a failure in the brain may also be small or large, affecting only one connection or several connections allowing us to walk, talk, see, eat, and perform any of the innumerable functions that are a part of our daily lives—from blinking our eyelids to enjoying a good meal.

Of course, in the case of the body, the "shorting" of the brain is more complex than the shorting of a switchboard. Nerves carrying impulses to and from the brain are like wires, with the arteries providing power to the brain through blood containing glucose and oxygen supplies. A stroke, although it affects the nervous system, is due to a disturbance in the circulatory system of the brain. The disturbance can occur in one of three ways: A plug can build up in selected places in the arteries, causing a thrombus (plug), or the plug, instead of being stationary, can travel about the arteries until this plug (embolus) finally lands at a particular site; or there may be a weakness in the wall of the artery, causing the artery to rupture and resulting in a hemorrhage. The final result is the same—damage to a particular area of the brain.

The most common cause of stroke is due to a stationary plug or a narrowing in an artery to the brain. The process that most often initiates this is atherosclerosis, hardening of the arteries. Hardening of the arteries causes narrowing of the arteries and thrombosis, and the process can involve arteries in the neck or in the brain, or both.

Before going into detail on the anatomy of a stroke and the several causes, there are certain general points that can be made about the results of a stroke:

1. If one side of the brain is injured, the opposite side of the body will be affected. If the stroke is on the right side of the brain, the left side of the body will be affected.

2. The loss of function or paralysis depends on the site of the brain damage *and* on the extent. The extent may mean the loss of only one function—or it may be so great that so much of the brain is deprived of its vital blood, glucose, and oxygen that the body is unable to function enough to live. *Most strokes affect only relatively small areas of the brain.*

3. If a person is right-handed, the left hemisphere of the brain is dominant. The dominant side of the brain is also the side that controls speech. (Recent studies show that language centers are located in the left side of the brain in 97 percent of the population, but 89 percent of us are right-handed. This means that the language center is on the right in only three percent of the population, although 11 percent of us are left-handed. The result is that some left-handed people do have left-hemisphere dominance.) From what we know, however, if the left side of the brain is damaged and the person is right-handed, we may assume that the damage may cause speech impairment, known as *aphasia,* as well as paralysis. If the nondominant side of the brain is involved, there will be paralysis but no speech impairment, which was what happened after Louis Pasteur's first stroke—an artery on the right side of the brain was involved, paralyzing his left side, but not interfering with his speech.

Circulation in the Neck

Blood is supplied to the brain by four principal arteries that come from the area of the heart and go through the neck to reach the brain. People who have devoted themselves to the study of strokes feel that many strokes are the result of the interference with blood in the arteries in the neck going *to* the brain.

Think about this for a minute, and it makes sense.

There are four arteries that go through the neck in order to reach the brain. The two arteries in the front of the neck are the right and left internal carotid arteries. The two arteries in the back of the neck, near the spine, are called the vertebral arteries. These four arteries join together at the base of the brain in what is known as the Circle of Willis, since they form a kind of circle and Willis first described it. This "circle" gives off branches supplying blood to all areas of the brain.

The carotid (neck) arteries are subject to hardening of the arteries and may become narrowed or have their openings obliterated, or both. If this occurs predominantly on one side, a stroke may occur, with paralysis on the opposite side of the body (*hemiplegia,* or loss of function on one side, involves the upper and lower extremities on the same side of the body). To repeat, if

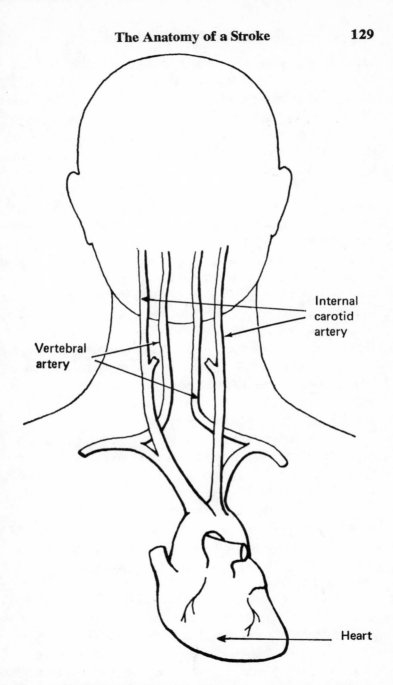

FIG. 5 LIFELINES (ARTERIES) THROUGH NECK TO BRAIN

the right side of the brain is injured, the left half of the body will be affected and vice versa.

So, if the right carotid artery in the neck is obstructed, a left-sided hemiplegia will occur. The arteries *within* the brain were not obstructed and did not cause the stroke; the injury to the artery in the *neck* set up the stroke and affected the brain.

In order to test whether the arteries in the neck are open, the physician or neurologist will compare the force of the beat on both sides of the neck. He will also listen with the stethoscope to find out if the beat on either side is accompanied by a noise called a *bruit*. This noise is akin to the sound produced by blowing over a narrowed bottle top. It suggests a narrowed artery.

Another method of checking the arteries may require the skills of an ophthalmologist (a physician who treats the eye and eye diseases). How is this done?

The internal carotid (neck) artery gives off only one branch in the neck that can be indirectly measured. This branch is called the ophthalmic artery and, as its name implies, it goes to the eye.

By measuring the pressure in the ophthalmic artery, we have an index of pressure in the carotid artery. The measurement of the pressure in both eyes is called (hold your breath!) *ophthalmodynamometry* (ODM).

If a person with stroke warning signs has a *decreased pulsation* in the carotid artery, along with a *bruit,* and has ODM findings indicating a decreased pressure in that artery, special *X-ray studies* are called for. This is done by a method called *arteriography*.

X-ray dye (actually an organic iodide that is opaque to X-rays) is injected into the arterial system and X-ray pictures are taken of the arteries of the neck and brain. The demonstration of narrowing or obstruction of the arteries of the brain often requires the specialized skills of the *neuroradiologist* (X-ray specialist dealing with

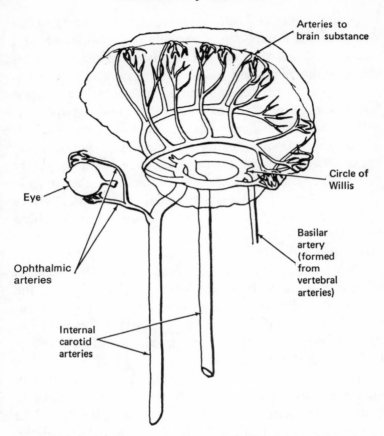

Arteries to
brain substance

Circle of
Willis

Eye

Basilar
artery
(formed
from
vertebral
arteries)

Ophthalmic
arteries

Internal
carotid
arteries

FIG. 6 CIRCULATION TO BRAIN AND EYE. PRESSURE MEASUREMENT
IN OPHTHALMIC ARTERY REFLECTS PRESSURE IN INTERNAL
CAROTID ARTERY

the brain and nervous system). If the arteriogram confirms the presence of a narrowing or obstruction of the carotid artery, and the obstruction or narrowing is surgically repaired, a full-fledged stroke may be avoided. Treatment with anticlotting medication can also be effective, and this may be the treatment of choice.

Mrs. D.H.'s case is typical of how this examination can save lives. She is a 52-year-old, heavy-smoking mother of two grown children. She returned to college to complete her training in accountancy after the children had left home. While cooking dinner one evening, she noticed that she couldn't stir the soup she was heating. Her left hand and forearm were numb. The vision in her right eye faded momentarily. The entire episode lasted about one minute. Mrs. D.H. reported the episode to her physician, whose examination was supplemented by ODM and arteriography. A severe narrowing of the right carotid artery was found and surgically corrected. Mrs. D.H. has now completed the courses she needs for her college degree and has a fruitful life to look forward to. She has stopped smoking, is watching her diet, and feels fine now.

Arteries of the Brain

Despite the importance of the neck arteries as causes of stroke, strokes also occur if the arteries that form the Circle of Willis and branch off into the brain are involved. What happened to Mrs. L.C. is somewhat typical, although she had no warning of impending cerebrovascular insult (stroke).

Mrs. L.C. is in her 50s. The day before her stroke, she was perfectly healthy. She did her housework, called her married daughter in Kansas City, wrote to her son in college, and fixed dinner for her husband and herself. The couple watched television afterward, and she read a bit before going to bed at her usual time. In the morning, when she awakened, she was partially paralyzed. Within a short time, she couldn't speak. Her doctor advised hospitalization.

Why did she have this stroke?

We *do* know that basically there was a decrease in the blood supplied to Mrs. L.C.'s brain that caused her stroke, and that she had this stroke because of underlying hardening of the arteries going to the brain. Under normal conditions, the brain requires a great deal of oxygen and glucose to function properly. Blood containing

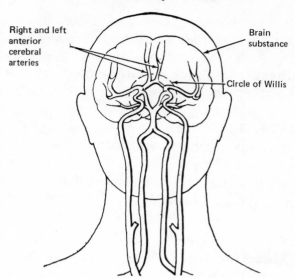

FIG. 7 ILLUSTRATION OF STROKE DUE TO OBSTRUCTION OF ANTERIOR CEREBRAL ARTERY

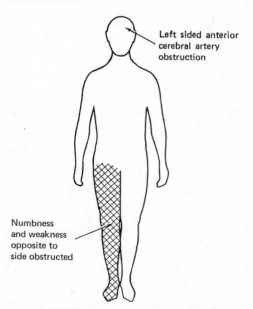

LEFT-SIDED OBSTRUCTION CAUSES RIGHT LOWER EXTREMITY DISABILITY

glucose is brought to the brain continuously through the arterial system. Any time that there is a reduction of the blood flow to the brain, oxygen deprivation with consequent brain damage may follow. Sometimes a sudden fall in blood pressure can give rise to stroke symptoms. In any case, if the oxygen and glucose supply fails only momentarily, the injury to the nerve cells may be transient and the disability will disappear. If the deprivation occurs over a prolonged period of time (measured in minutes), nerve cells may die, causing different sorts of disabilities that are technically called *neurological deficits*.

Mrs. L.C.'s stroke was due to hardening of the arteries, which had blocked an artery to the brain. In her case, the blockage occurred in one of the important arteries supplying blood and oxygen to a precise area of brain tissue, controlling specific functions of the body. The deprivation of oxygen and glucose resulted in specific neurological symptoms: paralysis and aphasia. There could have been other symptoms as well.

We mentioned earlier the carotid and vertebral arteries of the neck and how they join in the Circle of Willis. Other arteries branch upwards from the circle, carrying more blood, oxygen, and glucose into all areas of the brain. One of the arterial branches is the *anterior cerebral artery*. *Anterior* means "in front," and this artery serves the frontal area of the brain. Damage here, due to the interruption of the blood supply, results in impairment of the person's ability to move a leg or an arm, with loss of sensation in the leg.

Another artery is the *posterior cerebral artery* (in the rear of the brain). If this artery is blocked, the person may have visual difficulties because of damage to the visual cortex, the brain center controlling vision. Al-

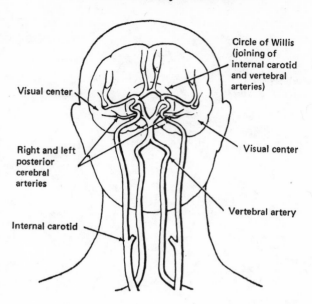

FIG. 8   ILLUSTRATION OF STROKE DUE TO OBSTRUCTION OF
POSTERIOR CEREBRAL ARTERY

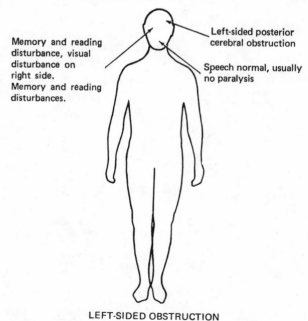

LEFT-SIDED OBSTRUCTION

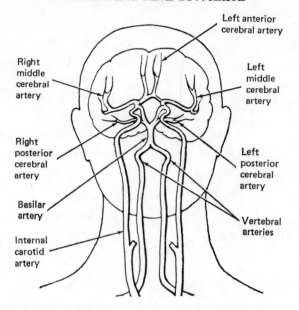

FIG. 9   ILLUSTRATION OF STROKE DUE TO OBSTRUCTION OF MIDDLE
          CEREBRAL ARTERY

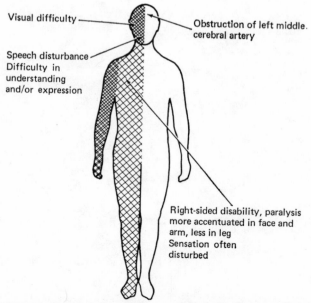

LEFT-SIDED OBSTRUCTION CAUSES RIGHT SIDED DISABILITY

though blindness can be total at the onset of the stroke, it usually regresses to the eye within hours.

The *middle cerebral artery* is one of the most common arteries involved in stroke. If the brain is damaged because of interruption of the blood flow here, the arm and leg and face may be partially or totally paralyzed on the side opposite to the side of the brain where the lesion occurs.

The basilar artery helps to form the Circle of Willis. It, in turn, is formed by the vertebral arteries.

Artery Affected	Symptoms
Posterior cerebral artery	Memory and reading disturbances, despite normal speech
	Vision defects on one side
Middle cerebral artery	Numbness and/or weakness more accentuated in face and arm area, less in lower limbs
	Visual difficulty
	Possible speech disturbances
Basilar artery	Vision difficulties
	Numbness in face or extremities
	Difficulty in swallowing, talking
	Many other symptoms, depending on size of involvement, such as unsteadiness, drowsiness, sudden collapse without loss of consciousness, or weakness in the extremities

Regardless of whether the stroke is ischemic, embolic

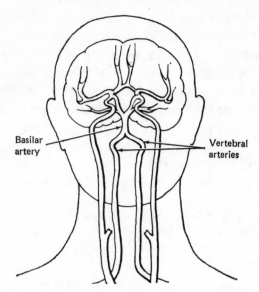

FIG. 10   ILLUSTRATION OF STROKE DUE TO OBSTRUCTION OF VERTEBROBASILAR ARTERY

Basilar artery

Vertebral arteries

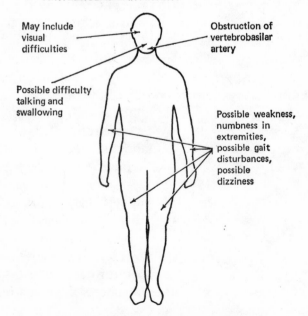

May include visual difficulties

Obstruction of vertebrobasilar artery

Possible difficulty talking and swallowing

Possible weakness, numbness in extremities, possible gait disturbances, possible dizziness

OBSTRUCTION OF BASILAR ARTERY
MAY CAUSE MANY SYMPTOMS

(thrombotic), or due to a cerebral hemorrhage (Chapter I), the results of the stroke will be similar, depending on the area of the brain affected. The "warning sign of stroke" that has been mentioned before, the transient ischemic attack (TIA), may also result in similar disabilities or neurological deficits, depending on what part of the brain is deprived of oxygen. There is a difference, however.

Transient Ischemic Attacks

A transient ischemic attack is a brief episode of neurological deficit, usually lasting a few seconds to a few hours. The episodes themselves are usually stereotyped. They can be severe, causing the appearance of hemiplegia or aphasia, and they may occur with considerable frequency. Some patients report 5 or even 20 a day. They may also be so mild or transient that the person is unaware he has had an attack or episode. All functions generally return to normal between attacks.

The attacks are usually thought to be warnings of impending neurological *disaster*—a stroke, in brief. Of 100 patients with TIA, at least 35 percent will develop a complete stroke within five years, and some experts estimate that the incidence is as high as 50 percent. Thus every patient with transient cerebral ischemia must be regarded as stroke-prone and treated to prevent catastrophe. Sometimes surgery may reduce the chance of stroke. At other times an anticlotting medication may be prescribed to try to prevent clot formation. While these drugs, if used early enough, can reduce further TIA, it is also thought that they can lessen the chance of a complete stroke.

These attacks are most often associated with plaques of atherosclerosis in the neck (cervical) and brain (cerebral) arteries, the presumed mechanism being that bits of the plaque break off and plug smaller, distant arteries. A similar analogy is what happens in a car, if the fuel lines are dirty, not necessarily plugging the carburetor but causing the engine to miss.

Other and rarer causes of TIA may be arterial spasms, lowering of the blood pressure in a narrow artery, and compression of the vertebral arteries because of arthritis in the neck. If blood flow in the carotid arterial system is decreased, weakness of the arm and leg on one side of the body, alterations of sensations on one side of the body, incomplete vision in one eye, or difficulty in speaking may follow. If the blood flow in the vertebral-basilar system (see FIGURE 10) is disturbed, the common symptoms of TIA may include dizziness, weakness of one or two extremities, double vision, difficulty in swallowing, transient blindness, confusion, unconsciousness, and sudden fainting spells.

The symptoms are transient and may occur singly or in any combination.

TIA from disturbed blood flow through a carotid artery typically include the following symptoms:

1.   Visual difficulties in one eye
2.   Weakness or disturbances in sensation on the side opposite to the vision difficulty
3.   Speech difficulty

Symptoms of TIA arising from disturbed blood flow through the basilar artery include the following:

1.   Dizziness
2.   Double vision
3.   Difficulty with speech
4.   Loss of equilibrium
5.   Faintness

Dr. Walter C. Alvarez popularized the concept of the "little" or "silent" stroke. Dr. Alvarez feels that many strokes occur in the "silent" areas of the brain where they are overlooked because they don't produce sufficient signs. Changes in personality, mental acuity, loss of interest, and other nonspecific symptoms lead to difficulty in diagnosing the "little stroke." This concept is interesting and deserving of further supportive research.

Brain Hemorrhage

Brain hemorrhage, or bleeding into the brain, occurs in about 20 percent of all new strokes. Among the minor causes (from the point of view of statistics, not the patient) are head injuries, bleeding tendencies, and brain tumors. *Aneurysms* (bulges in the arterial wall) of a cerebral artery and congenital malformations (abnormalities we are born with) of the blood vessels of the brain may also cause cerebral hemorrhage. Prevention of brain bleeding due to some of these causes—for example malformations—are not possible at present. Nevertheless, they are treatable.

Although strokes are associated with apparently healthy persons of middle age, with the years of high productivity and family responsibility, they may also occur in younger people. This is often the case with congenital malformations.

Mr. A.B.C. is an engineer of 26. He was helping his wife with spring cleaning, when he suddenly cried out for help. By the time that his wife reached him, he was unconscious on the floor. He was taken to the hospital, where he regained consciousness but was confused and irrational, complaining of a severe frontal headache. After the appropriate tests were performed, his physicians determined that he had a congenital malformation of the blood vessels at the base of the brain. Surgery was performed, and Mr. A.B.C.'s recovery was complete and uneventful.

His case illustrates the treatability of just one cause of cerebral hemorrhage. Some of the causes listed above are not preventable. Suffering a head injury is usually beyond the limits of prevention, since its cause is generally innocently accidental. Bleeding tendencies may also be due to sensitivity to medications or due to diseases

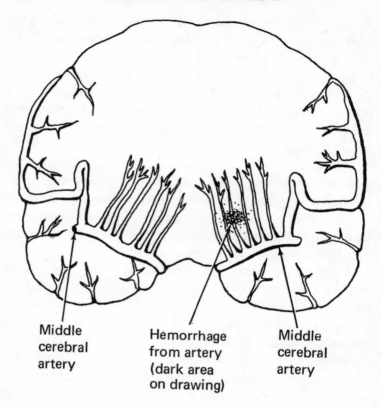

Middle cerebral artery

Hemorrhage from artery (dark area on drawing)

Middle cerebral artery

FIG. 11   A COMMON SITE OF BRAIN HEMORRHAGE

affecting our clotting mechanisms. These, too, are treatable.

High blood pressure is considered to be one of the most important factors in the production of cerebral hemorrhage. The evidence for this is considerable. Dr. Whisnant and his co-workers in Rochester, Minnesota, found that high blood pressure was present *before* the hemorrhage in 89 percent of patients with cerebral hemorrhage. The important Framingham study recorded a strong correlation between high blood pressure and stroke. These studies confirmed actuarial studies showing that high blood pressure increased the risk for all types of stroke. The Veterans Administration cooperative studies provide additional rationale for the treatment of high blood pressure to prevent cerebrovascular disease.

A much-feared form of bleeding is the *subarachnoid hemorrhage,* in which bleeding occurs into the space between two of the layers covering the brain.

This bleeding may be associated with aneurysms (weaknesses in the wall of the artery causing a bulge), which then go on to rupture. Another cause of this type of brain hemorrhage is the rare congenital arteriovenous (A-V) malformation that affects both arteries (arterio-) and veins (venous). One is born with this type of condition, and it is considered to be the result of a developmental error.

Aneurysms are more common. They generally occur in the medium-size arteries of the Circle of Willis, where the branches of the carotid artery join at the base of the brain. It used to be thought that brain aneurysms were congenital, but recent evidence indicates that there may be a relationship between sustained high blood pressure and large (or gross) aneurysms around the Circle of Willis.

Micro-, or tiny, aneurysms have been found in the small branches of the arteries forming the Circle of Willis. They have been observed as a result of the development of low-voltage X-ray techniques. If these tiny aneurysms rupture, they may cause strokes.

In either case, we think it may be reasonable to assume that effective control of blood pressure may prevent the development of aneurysms, either large or small. Such effective control of blood pressure in longstanding or severe high blood pressure disease may forestall the rupture of aneurysms that are already present by reducing the stress on the arterial walls.

Although surgery has been mentioned in the treatment of some types of stroke, surgery is possible only in certain instances. Moreover—and more important—surgery in any form cannot rejuvenate dead nerve tissue. Once a person has had a stroke, surgery cannot correct the disability due to the *death* of brain tissue.

The Stroke Syndrome

There are causes of stroke other than thrombosis, hemorrhage, and embolism—or the causes just mentioned, aneurysms and congenital arteriovenous malformations. These other causes are many. They result in similar damage to the brain, but are caused by different processes than true stroke (common or vascular stroke).

Some of the conditions that cause this stroke syndrome are given below. For example, a person with a brain tumor or brain abscess may appear similar to a person with a vascular stroke. One of the major problems to be sorted out by the physician is the precise cause of the stroke, so that the cause as well as the stroke itself can be treated. Was the stroke due to a brain tumor, for example? Or was it due to multiple sclerosis, an abscess, or other less common causes?

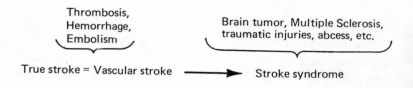

FIG. 12   CONDITION CAUSING STROKE SYNDROME

To help rule out these other possibilities, the attending physician and the neurologist will want as much of a detailed history of the onset of paralysis as possible. This history may frequently suggest vascular stroke as a likely diagnosis. If the onset is gradual, thrombosis is likely to be the cause. If both sides of the brain are affected simultaneously, however, so that the person is paralyzed on both sides, the paralysis is less likely to be due to a stroke. The answer to whether a person has had a vascular stroke is often far from simple. The history of the onset is usually not enough.

A thorough examination of the patient's nervous system and a thorough physical examination plus confirmatory laboratory tests are called for.

The anatomy of the brain and the blood vessels within the brain and those supplying it with blood, oxygen, and glucose is needed are beautifully ordered, each in relation to the others. To make sure of a completely accurate diagnosis and to pinpoint the exact area and cause of the stroke, the evaluating physician may need skull X rays, a lumbar puncture (spinal tap), a brain scan (radioactive survey of the brain), an electroencephalogram (brain-wave testing), and arteriography (X rays of the arteries of the brain).

While these tests are most useful in helping to confirm—or rule out—the usual causes of stroke, they also serve other purposes. The brain scan is a simple procedure, in which a minute amount of radioactive material is injected into a vein. The material concentrates itself in abnormal areas of the brain and then can show up as an exceptionally dense region on an image collected by a Geiger counter, an instrument used to measure radiation.

Still another, and a new, technique of brain-scanning evaluates the flow of blood to the brain, providing evidence of stroke through measuring the different cadence or rhythm of the flow as a result of the stroke, as opposed to the cadence of flow due to other causes. For example, the brain scan immediately following an ischemic stroke is normal. During the first 10 to 14 days after a stroke, it becomes abnormal. Then the abnormal area gradually fades, taking approximately two months to disappear. A brain tumor or other lesions of the brain have entirely different patterns.

The most sensitive and the most reliable diagnostic technique is the arteriogram. It carries more risk to the patient than the other techniques, so it is not used routinely. If the diagnosis is at all in question, however, an arteriogram is used because it actually allows the physicians to visualize the blood vessels of the brain and detect blockage or occlusion of specific blood vessels, tumors, blood clots on the surface of the brain as opposed to clots inside the arteries, abnormal blood vessels, and many other general disease processes.

The "Who" of Stroke

The cases described in this chapter and other chapters depict the wide variety of people who have had a stroke and what happens to them. Yet it should be kept in mind that everyone and anyone—including you and me—can have a stroke: Men and women, and children, too, regardless of the general association of stroke with the middle and later years of life, can have stroke. Even infants can have strokes. Thankfully, this is extremely rare.

Certain types of stroke and stroke syndromes seem to be associated with certain ages, however, and they have been classified as follows:

Infants (0 to 2 years old). The most common cause is the subdural hematoma, an encapsulated blood clot. Stroke may also be caused by a thrombosis (clot) or inflammation of a blood vessel of the brain, resulting in acute "infantile" hemiplegia, paralysis on one side.

Children (3 to 10 years old). Acute "infantile" hemiplegia may still occur during these years. Other causes are *venous sinus thrombosis,* a clot in the veins carrying blood from the brain; embolism; blood disorders; and high blood pressure that stems from nephritis (kidney disease).

Adolescents (10 to 20 years old). These are the ages between which a congenital aneurysm or vascular malformation may rupture, causing a cerebral hemorrhage. Another cause may be the result of embolism.

Young adults (20 to 35 years old). Again, congenital aneurysms or vascular malformations may rupture during these years, causing a stroke. Stroke syndrome may be a result of multiple sclerosis and tumors.

Middle-aged adults (35 to 60). These are the years during which people are most stroke-prone—the years of high productivity and family responsibility. Ruptured congenital aneurysms or vascular malformations may still cause strokes, but the most common cause are ischemia or thrombosis in the carotid arterial system and embolism. Subdural hematomas and tumors may also cause stroke syndrome.

Older adults (60 years old and older). Narrowing or thrombosis of the arteries supplying blood to the brain and cerebral hemorrhage are the major causes of stroke during these years.

We have examined the causes of true stroke and referred to other causes (stroke syndrome), as well as the causes that are more apt to affect people at different ages. The basic causes of thrombosis, hemorrhage, and embolism, however, are hardening of the arteries and sustained high blood pressure. There are many disease states and other factors that hasten or accelerate the development of hardening of the arteries and the elevating of blood pressure. Some of the disease states are diabetes, gout, disorders of fat metabolism, and heart disease. Some of the factors associated with stroke seem to be smoking, age, sex, race, heredity, geography, diet, oral contraceptives, weight, clotting factors in the blood, and stress.

The combination of factors that predispose a person to stroke is referred to as a prestroke profile. As we gather more knowledge about who gets stroke and who doesn't, the prestroke profile will become more and more sophisticated. In the meantime, we must rely on, and act upon, what we know about preventing strokes. We know much. We can do much.

CHAPTER IX

STROKE AND REHABILITATION

The specialty of rehabilitation medicine (physiatry) attained official recognition in 1947. Since that time, this specialty has become a vital part of the comprehensive care of most patients, including the stroke patient. Indeed, most of the time necessary to restore a patient after a stroke so he can return to an active daily life is done under the supervision of, or by, the "physical medicine" specialist—the physiatrist.

The recovery of complete function in the patient who has suffered weakness or paralysis of one half of the body (hemiplegia) depends on the extent of the damage produced by the clot, hemorrhage, or embolus that affected the artery to the brain. If the extent of the brain damage is extensive, functional improvement will take more time and effort. In patients with hemorrhage into the brain substance itself, active rehabilitation measures are postponed until the condition of the patient has stabilized. In all cases, nevertheless, the aim is to start rehabilitation therapy as soon after the stroke as possible.

The concurrent medical management of assorted and associated illnesses goes on throughout the recovery period and subsequently for life. Associated heart disease, high blood pressure, or diabetes, which may affect the pace or tempo of rehabilitation, is carefully evaluated, monitored, and treated.

Family and friends should be included in the rehabilitative process for psychological support and for very practical purposes. It is unfortunate but true that complications seemingly occur more on weekends than during the week. Weekend diseases are linked with reduced staff and reduced observation. It is during these times that patients occasionally become dehydrated, or their diabetes goes awry, or their heart disease associated with the stroke may not be so closely monitored. It is on weekends that the training program ceases. So it is on weekends that family and friends can be of special assistance—of course, with the specific approval of the hospital staff. The staff is often eager to enlist the assistance of cooperative volunteers to help with training.

The stroke victim is more than fortunate if his family and his friends become actively involved in the process of rehabilitation. The frequent depressions that occur after stroke respond better to the tender, loving care of family and friends than to drugs. The feeling of desperation that may arise in a patient who can't speak usually improves with time, training, and the interest of the family and hospital staff. By the same token, as the patient improves the family is encouraged and time helps heal the wounds of both the patient and the loved ones.

An enemy to recovery is fear. For example, fear often inhibits and delays the return of a stroke victim's sexual activity, but people who have had a stroke can and do return to their customary sexual pattern upon recovery. Understanding the fear by the non-affected husband or wife will help lessen the anxiety of the stroke victim. The resumption of sexual relations is valuable from the psychological point of view. The benefits include the rebuilding of confidence, release of tensions, and a resumption of pleasurable, warm personal feelings.

The preliminaries to sexual intercourse should not be forgotten. Time should be devoted to allow for sufficient excitation and play of both partners. The mind and the body need to be stirred gently in prelude to sexual intercourse. There is no one "normal" position in sexual intercourse. The best normal position is the one that the partners find physically satisfactory. The frequency of sexual intercourse varies greatly. It depends on the mental attitude and physical ability of the stroke victim. Fatigue and physical exhaustion pose the outstanding limitations to sex in the recovered stroke victim.

Problems of Rehabilitation

The major problem of the stroke victim is to regain his sense of usefulness and independence. This is achieved by repetitive training preparing the patient for the activities of daily life. The restoration of the stroke victim to self-sufficiency in the shortest possible time is the goal of this team effort. Some of the special problems are:

The painful shoulder. During the state of paralysis, the weight of the arm causes pulling on the shoulder joint. Propping the arm on a pillow and using a simple sling can help avoid the pulling weight of this limb on the shoulder.

Pain about the shoulder can also be due to a fall that may have occurred at the time of the stroke, and fractures of the shoulder may be the cause of such pain. Most shoulder pain, however, is due simply to not enough early exercising of the arm after stroke. When the shoulder is not assisted in exercises, the muscles about it may contract and the result is pain when the arm is moved. Occasionally, a stroke victim will have pain about the shoulder *and* pain in the hand. This so-called hand-shoulder problem (syndrome) happens sometimes after both heart attacks and strokes. The reasons aren't quite clear. Special treatments are required.

A "Helping Hand." If the hand is contracted so that the nails tend to dig into the palm, simple measures such as cutting the nails of the paralyzed hand can avoid trouble. Exercising the hand by moving the fingers and wrist may help prevent painful swelling and ease contraction of the hand. Routine splinting of the arm is now frowned upon by most physiatrists. They generally advocate assisted (passive) exercise and gradually unassisted (active) exercise to prevent complications. The hand may be the last extremity to recover.

The lower extremities. In the usual stroke, the paralysis of the leg usually recedes before that of the arm. The ability to sit, stand, and then walk, however, requires progressive instructions to develop the necessary balance and motor power. Walking is taught with the assistance of a "walker" or parallel bar, or both. As ability increases, fear decreases and learning in the other activities of daily living proceeds. The use of a leg brace to help the foot and ankle is quite common. Most hemiplegic patients can be sucessfully taught to walk.

Speech disorders. One of the most common problems of stroke are speech disorders (aphasia). Aphasia is most usual when the brain injury involves the dominant side of the brain—that is, the left side of the brain in a naturally right-handed individual. When a person can't write as well as speak, it is called *expressive,* or *motor, aphasia.* When the patient cannot understand what is said or what he reads, the aphasia is called *receptive,* or *sensory, aphasia.* Therapy is possible and can be effective. The process is often long and time-consuming, requiring patience on the part of both the stroke victim and family.

Perceptual difficulties. Depending on the part of the brain involved, the victim of a stroke may have loss of sight in one eye or in a field of vision. A person may see straight ahead out of his right eye but not to the right side, for example. This means that the person may have difficulty in getting his hand to his mouth so he can eat by himself. He may also have difficulty in seeing on one side. Depth perception may be awry. Therapy, again, can help train the stroke victim to adapt to these perceptual difficulties.

The process of recovery from a stroke is slow and difficult. It is often marred by frustration and anxiety to both the patient and the family, but time, training, and understanding help make a difficult task somewhat easier.

Just as there are many specialized problems requiring specialized care in the stroke victim, there are specialized aids, too. There are combination knife and fork sets that can be used with one hand. There are elastic shoelaces, which make getting in and out of shoes easy, without the victim's needing to tie knots. There are shoehorns with long handles or on long sticks. There are bathtub seats for bathing, and raised adjustable toilet seats that are of real practical value. There are three or four-legged canes, which provide more support than the conventional cane. However helpful these aids are, nothing has been invented or will be invented that will substitute for determination, hard work, and practice.

PART TWO:

STROKE AND PREVENTION

How can we retard or even reverse hardening of the arteries? What can we do about high blood pressure? How can we eat better and stop smoking so we can live longer, healthier lives—and hopefully prevent a stroke or heart attack?

If a stroke or heart trouble cannot be completely prevented, we still can do a lot to *lower* the risks. Some of the answers to these questions involve the help of your physician. Many of the suggestions depend on you and your desire for life.

CHAPTER X

DIET—LOWERING THE TABLE STAKES

Gambling can be dangerous. Gambling with your life can be deadly. With respect to stroke and heart disease, you are really dealing with "table stakes" when it comes to the steaks *on* the table—and you may be "buttering" up the odds stacked against you, if you eat improperly.

One steak and one pat of butter alone won't cause a stroke, of course. But we are often our own worst enemies, and stroke is a perfect example. Medicine offers no magic pill, no abracadabra prescription, and no easy way to prevent stroke, although it does offer an effective, common-sense preventive program to reduce the table stakes and the odds. The prudent diet is part of the program.

As long as a person "feels good," however, the average American sees little reason to worry about hardening of the arteries or high blood pressure, two major causes of stroke, or to give up steaks. It's all too easy for many people to ignore what is happening within their bodies until it is too late to prevent the 200,000 strokes, apart from the heart attacks, that suddenly strike Americans each year.

At least *some* of those 200,000 Americans could have avoided the strokes that killed or crippled them. Stroke does not have to be inevitable and, in some cases, it is preventable. For one thing, many people—unwittingly—go to great lengths to increase their chances of having a stroke. They are playing against loaded dice. Eventually they will lose.

Average Americans of their own free will eat too many rich foods, which not only lead to overweight but perhaps to high cholesterol levels and hardening of the arteries—and finally to stroke and heart trouble.

In an effort to avoid the unpleasantness of giving up something they like, some people seek a rationale, an excuse, especially if it is in the guise of a "scientific fact." One that popped up a few years ago was that eggs contain lecithin. Lecithin, it was said, offset the cholesterol in egg yolks. Thus, the standard, old-fashioned American breakfast of bacon or ham and eggs was all right to eat.

The fact is: Eggs do contain lecithin, but lecithin does *not* protect against fats in the diet.

Two eggs contain 500 milligrams of cholesterol. These 500 milligrams of cholesterol can potentially raise a person's blood cholesterol level about 25 to 30 points, according to Dr. Jean Mayer, noted Harvard nutritionist. That 25 or 30 milligrams can elevate a "safe" cholesterol level of 180 or 200 to well above the risk level—and the person still has not eaten all the cholesterol-containing food that he most likely will eat the rest of the day.

It is not the eggs one or two days a week that will materially damage our arteries, but it is the constant breakfast diet of eggs and all the lunches and dinners that rely on meats rich in cholesterol and saturated fats, plus the fat-rich dairy products.

Stroke and heart disease are not the only diseases that strike home through the kitchen as far as food preferences and misinformation are concerned. Cardiovascular disease has been more closely associated in the public's mind with food than have many other diseases, although cancer has come in for its share of jumping-

on-the-bandwagon of unproven facts, too. Unproven
observations or interesting sidelights tend to be picked
up, rather than actual facts.

An English cancer team recently disturbed coffee lov-
ers by noting in one study that persons who drank large
amounts of coffee had more cancer than those who
drank little coffee. Others have associated coffee with
heart disease. Is it true? Probably not. It has yet to be
confirmed by a controlled study. Other researchers a
few years ago found that churchgoers had more strokes
and heart trouble than nonchurchgoers. No one seriously suggested that people give up going to church. Studies of this sort are poorly controlled, announced pre-
maturely in the media as fact, and are generally proven
to be erroneous later on. There is enough known and
proven to the satisfaction of most physicians about the
relationship between stroke and heart disease and food
without searching for a link that is probably coincidental.

Low-cholesterol foods, free of saturated fat, do not
have to be punishment, just to prove how good they are
for you. There are ways to make any diet enjoyable
without having it taste bad, especially when the reward
is good health.

No diet, nevertheless, is a substitute for regular medical checkups, including periodic checks of blood fats
and blood pressure. The attitude that "what you don't
know won't hurt you" can not only hurt but even kill
you if it produces a stroke or a heart attack.

The Prudent Diet

A prudent diet does not mean giving up everything a
person likes. You may still eat your steak or your bacon
and eggs—as long as you don't eat them every day.
Gourmet dishes are not out either; there are substitutes
for the cream and eggs in many of the sauces, which reduce the saturated-fat and cholesterol content without

distracting from the taste. Aside from substituting some foods or ingredients for others, however, many of the principles of a prudent diet may already be familiar if you learn a little about the basic elements of good nutrition.

The prudent diet recommended to prevent hardening of the arteries is not a weight-losing diet. It may help control weight, however, for those who want to maintain a desirable weight or have already lost weight.

Prudent-diet meal planning follows the basic rules for minimum daily requirements of protein, carbohydrates, vitamins, minerals, and fat (polyunsaturated only) that are included in any good, healthful diet. The result is that many of these rules should be familiar to women, who as wives and mothers bear the responsibility for food shopping and menu planning and cooking. Since men are more susceptible to hardening of the arteries, stroke, and heart trouble, they too should raise their levels of awareness and understanding about foods.

The following rules and tables are based on *The Prudent Diet,* a publication of the New York City Health Services Administration, revised in 1972. In your prudent diet be sure to:

1. Include vegetables and fruit that are high in minerals and vitamins and low in fat and calories. Most, if not all, of these are cholesterol-free, so you can eat them to your cardiovascular content.

2. Include bread and unsweetened cereals. Eaten in moderation, these are low in fat, unfattening, and contain essential nutrition. More, later, on the milk to top the cereal.

3. Include a high-quality protein in each meal. This means avoiding the so-called red meats as much as possible in favor of fish, lean meats,

poultry, and low-fat cheeses. Any beef should be lean, with the fat removed before cooking, and broiled to cut down on the saturated fats. Eggs may be eaten, but no more than four a week, *including* any eggs used in cooking and baking. Vegetable and cereal foods (dried beans, peas, nuts) contain adequate protein, fewer calories, less saturated fat, and can be combined with a small amount of animal protein to make delicious meals, low in cholesterol.

4. Include unsaturated and polyunsaturated fats, including oils and margarines, rather than saturated fats (butter) and cooking fats.

5. Limit those empty calories in candy, soft drinks, cakes, pies, and pastry. For home-baked foods, use unsaturated fats, rather than conventional saturated ones.

6. Eat three meals a day for better control of your appetite, more efficient use of foods, and less temptation to snack and increase weight.

7. Maintain a desirable weight. This means, if you're overweight, that you should reduce with the help of your physician. Remember, your food requirements change with age. If you're between 35 and 55, you should reduce your total caloric intake 5 percent for each ten years. If you're between 55 and 75, reduce it 8 percent for each decade.

These are the seven basic rules for eating well and preventing heart disease and stroke. They take into account a balanced diet, meeting the daily minimum requirements for all nutrients, including protein, vitamins, and minerals. While the rules limit the *total* fat content, they do provide for a desirable ratio of *polyunsaturated* to saturated fat.

Here is how the recommended foods, and those to avoid as much as possible, tie in with the basic nutritional food groups. (See opposite page.)

The Prudent Diet

Food Groups	Foods Recommended	Foods to Avoid or Use Seldom
VEGETABLES AND FRUITS Supply vitamins, minerals and calories.	*Eat vegetables daily*—cooked, raw, fresh, frozen, canned.	
Furnish vitamin C and iron when properly prepared.	Eat vegetables high in vitamin A 4 or 5 times a week.	
	Dark green leafy—broccoli, kale, spinach greens, collard, mustard, turnip greens	
	Deep yellow—carrots, pumpkin, sweet potatoes, winter squash	
	Potatoes and a variety of other vegetables provide additional vitamins and minerals.	
Supply vitamin C.	*Eat fruits daily.*	Avocado—high in fat
	Eat daily grapefruit, oranges, tangerines, tomatoes, cantaloupes, strawberries, mango, papaya.	
	A variety of other fruits provide additional vitamins and minerals.	

ENRICHED AND WHOLE GRAIN BREADS OR CEREALS Supply B vitamins, iron, protein and calories.	*Eat breads or cereals daily.*	Baked products made with shortening or saturated fat— Muffins Biscuits Danish pastry Cookies Doughnuts Cakes and pies
MILK AND MILK PRODUCTS Supply high-quality protein, calcium, riboflavin and calories. Nonfat milk contains all the nutrients in whole milk except most of the fat.	*Drink milk daily.* 2 cups nonfat (skim) milk for adults 2 to 4 cups milk for children—some of this may be nonfat or low fat Include buttermilk, low fat milk, yogurt, evaporated skim milk. These contain about 1 percent butterfat. Choose nonfat dry milks with added vitamins A and D. Eat cheeses that are low in fat and high in protein: cottage, pot, farmer, imitation process cheese spread (fat content not more than 5 percent).	Whole milk—butterfat about 3½ per cent Cream—sweet, sour Milk puddings Ice cream Butter Cream cheese Cheese—made from whole milk Non-dairy cream substitutes High fat cheese—cheddar, swiss and dessert types

FISH, MEAT POULTRY, EGGS
Supply high-quality protein, iron, B vitamins and calories.

High in iron, Vitamin A and other vitamins.

Supply iron, B vitamins, calories, but not as high in protein as fish, meat, poultry and eggs.

Eat fish 4 or 5 times a week—for breakfast, lunch and dinner.

Eat chicken, turkey, lean veal often (lower in fat than beef, pork, lamb).

Lean beef, lean lamb, lean pork: limit to 3—4 servings a week (one serving is 4 oz. cooked—allow ⅓ pound raw of boneless or ½ pound raw meat with bones).

Liver—eat rarely.

Remove all visible fat from meat.

Shellfish—use rarely (high in cholesterol).

Eggs—2 a week for adults, 4 to 6 a week for children (yolk is high in cholesterol).

Dried beans and peas and nuts—use occasionally.

Select lean cuts of meat—beef: round, sirloin tip, rump; lamb: leg; pork: loin, ham or leg.

Chill soups and drippings to remove fat.

Duck
Goose
Organ meats:
Kidney
Brain
Sweetbreads
Fat Meats:
Bacon
Sausage
Corned beef
Pastrami
Salami
Frankfurters
Luncheon meats
Spareribs
Pigs' feet

FATS, VEGETABLE OILS AND SELECTED MARGARINES
Supply polyunsaturated fats and calories.

Use vegetable oils daily—2 to 3 tablespoons (1-1½ oz). for salads and in cooking.

Use corn, safflower, soybean, cottonseed oil (peanut oil is not polyunsaturated to the same degree).

Selected margarines—those that mention vegetable oil as first ingredient on label (ingredients are listed in order of quantity, so acceptable margarine *must list liquid vegetable oil first*).

Baked products made at home with vegetable oil or margarine with a substantial amount of liquid vegetable oil (see recipes in this booklet).

Do Not Gain Weight

Coconut oil
Olive oil
Animal fats:
   Lard
   Salt pork
   Fat back
   Butter
   Suet
Vegetable shortenings—
   artificially hardened
   (hydrogenated)
Baked products
   made with saturated
   fat or shortening—
   cakes, pies, cookies

Fats and Oils

Fats and oils bear special attention, since fats are the largest single donor of calories, regardless of whether they are saturated or unsaturated. Because of this, you might think of fats as being "visible" and "invisible." If you can see the fat—chicken fat, suet, lard, margarine, butter, salad oils—it's visible. The invisible fats are those in meats and in many commercial baked goods. The majority of the fats in most diets are the ones that are *invisible,* so the caloric (and cholesterol) values go uncounted. All in all, 50 percent of all calories come from these invisible fats. For example, one cup of *whole* milk has 170 calories in comparison to 85 calories for one cup of *nonfat* milk. Cakes and pies also have about 50 percent of their calories in fats—and most of these are saturated fats.

Because so many foods are "overweight" with fats, it can't be repeated often enough that fats are divided into three types: Saturated, or fats that are solid at room temperature, with the exception of coconut oil; unsaturated or polyunsaturated, that are liquid at room temperature; and monosaturated, olive and peanut oils that have little effect on cholesterol levels but may aggravate lesions due to hardening of the arteries.

To help you avoid the saturated fats that can raise cholesterol levels, here is a table of the most popular foods divided into categories, depending on the type of fat. If the list seems restrictive, remember the fact that a food is high in saturated fat or cholesterol does not mean it must be shunned forever in all forms—but it should be avoided as much as possible, and maybe even a little more than seems possible at first.

Fats and Foods

Predominantly saturated fat. Avoid or eat sparingly. The list includes products made from or with these foods, such as most cakes, pastry, cookies, gravy, sauces, and many snack foods.

Beef, veal, lamb, pork, and their products, such as cold cuts and sausages—all are predominantly saturated. Veal fat (veal is, after all, young beef) is predominantly saturated, as are the following items:

Eggs
Whole milk
Whole milk cheeses
Cream, both sweet and sour
Ice cream
Lard
Hydrogenated shortenings
Chocolate
Coconut

Predominantly polyunsaturated fats. Rely on these to lower cholesterol. They include the products made from and with them.

Liquid vegetable oils, such as corn, cottonseed, safflower, and soybean oils
Margarines containing substantial amounts of the oils above in liquid form
Fish
Nuts, such as walnuts, filberts, pecans, almonds
Poultry—chicken and turkey fat is more favorably distributed between polyunsaturated and satu‑ rated fats than is fat in red meats

Predominantly monosaturated fats. These have no ef‑ fect on raising cholesterol. At the same time, they should be eaten with discretion.

Olives
Olive oil
Avocadoes
Cashew nuts

Substituting Good for Bad

Some forms of a food may be low in fat and/or cho‑

lesterol, either because the forbidden element is separated by hand at home or because the food has been processed in a way that it is eliminated.

Eggs are a perfect example of the possibility of separating the offending cholesterol. Keep in mind that the *whites* of eggs, which are an excellent source of protein, can be eaten in quantity. Anyone, even a person in the high-risk group, can enjoy as many scrambled eggs as he wants as long as the 250 milligrams of cholesterol per yolk aren't there.

Scrambled eggs without yolks? Try them.

Simply separate the whites into a bowl, adding seasonings (salt, pepper, a drop of Worcestershire sauce), some skim milk, and a drop of yellow food coloring. Beat well and pour into a frying pan with unsaturated oil or margarine, cooking as usual. A new preparation takes even this work out of making noncholesterol scrambled eggs. It's called *Egg Beaters* and can be used in any recipe calling for eggs—except sunnyside up.

You can enjoy "sausage" or "ham," too, with textured vegetable protein breakfast sausage or ham. Made with soybeans basically, the products have the taste and texture of the natural meat—without the cholesterol or saturated fat. Miles Laboratories' Morningstar Farms is one brand to look for. A breading product for chicken, again low fat, is Adolph's *Gold 'n Crust*.

Milk and milk products are examples of foods in which the saturated fat can be removed. Cream, obviously, is banned from any prudent diet because of its high butterfat content. Whole milk and milk products (cheese) are also high on the forbidden list. The milk to be avoided even includes milks labeled "low-fat," which are actually a mixture of whole and skim milk, and "filled milks," since these are a combination of skim milk and vegetable oil, all too often coconut or hydrogenated oil.

This still leaves skim milk, canned evaporated skim milk, or powdered skim milk, all containing essentially no butterfat. These milks are invaluable in a low-saturated-fat, low-cholesterol diet. They can be drunk and they can be used in sauces and toppings. Powdered buttermilk is economical and handy, too, but it should be used only if the label reads "less than one percent butterfat." A powdered skim-milk buttermilk is on its way to the market, and it will be safe in any amount, just like powdered skim milk.

Milk is worth a special note for another reason. If you have young children in the family, you may feel they should drink whole milk, which contains nutrients they need—unless your physician prefers them to drink skim milk for special reasons. If there is a history of heart disease or stroke in the family or if the family is one that has high blood fats in it, it may be advisable to limit the cholesterol and fat intake *even in children.* This is the trend today and involves what has been termed the "Children's Crusade." Skim milk instead of whole milk and other dietary restrictions as well should be observed and followed to reduce fat intake.

With the exception of the milk and eggs that youngsters may also eat in larger quantities than adults, all the other rules and elements of the prudent diet pertain to them as well as to adults. In fact, learning to eat prudently when they're young may save them from hardening of the arteries and stroke and heart trouble in adulthood for two reasons: First, we think their arteries will be healthier, with fewer cholesterol deposits, and second, the food habits they learn when young won't have to be changed as they grow older.

Cheese is usually high in butterfat because of the whole milk used to make it. There are skim-milk cheeses, although they are generally made in foreign countries and are hard to find in this country. Then, too, they vary in fat content. Most cheese, therefore, is on the list of forbidden foods or foods to be eaten rarely. On the way to the market, however, are low-calorie, low-fat cheeses. The Fisher Cheese Company in Wapakoneta, Ohio, has such cheeses, which can be ordered by mail.

The one commercial cheese that can be eaten frequently is cottage cheese. Cottage cheese curd is made from skim milk and contains essentially no fat or cholesterol. Beware, though, of *creamed* cottage cheese, which has a high butterfat content, and "low-fat" cottage cheese that contains less cream than creamed cottage cheese but has some milk. If only creamed cottage cheese is available, it can be used—as long as the cream and milk are washed off.

Misconceptions About Food

Some of the misconceptions about food are already obvious. It isn't the number of calories that are eaten that count, for one. Important, too, is the source of those calories. If they are derived from fat and cholesterol, these calories are doubly dangerous.

Other misconceptions extend into the area of food products. For example, buying a powdered, nondairy cream substitute for use in coffee or tea is not the same as buying powdered skim milk. Many of these substitutes are made with coconut oil, rich in the saturated fat that produces hardening of the arteries at a much more rapid rate in experimental animals than unsaturated fats. The ice milk and sherbet that are often acceptable on a weight-losing diet because they are low in calories may be high in saturated fat. They may even have extra fat added, especially in the form of that dangerous and pervasive coconut oil. Good, low-fat ice cream is on its way to the market, however.

In addition, the fact that an item is "dried" doesn't mean that cholesterol has been "dried out" or removed.

Egg yolk in any form—fresh, frozen, or dried—is cholesterol rich. Egg yolks are ingredients in ice cream; cake, pancake, and waffle mixes; baked goods, egg noodles, canned soups, and some salad dressings. In other words, the only way to be sure of what you're eating is to read the label. Even then, it may be necessary at times to ask or write the manufacturer for a complete list of the product's contents. As of December 1973, however, manufacturers are required to list ingredients on the label, under federal law. This includes labeling for cholesterol, fats, and fatty acids, with the cholesterol stated in milligrams per serving and in milligrams per 100 grams (100 grams is a little more than 3 ounces). Fats and fatty acids will be listed similarly.

The list of ingredients in food is in order of their predominance in the product, with the ones listed first present in the greatest quantity by weight. In the case of margarine, manufacturers often partially hydrogenate the fat so that "partially hydrogenated" or "partially hardened" appears in the prime position. Hydrogenation is a process. It has nothing to do with whether a fat is originally saturated or polyunsaturated—any liquid oil can be "hardened" to give the oil more thickness, like butter. But hydrogenation does take the "polyun" out, so that hydrogenated fats are saturated. Soft or tub margarines, because of the quality of the fat, are usually the most highly polyunsaturated and are best.

The term *vegetable oil* is also ambiguous. Often it may be a combination of saturated and unsaturated oils, and terms like "hydrogenated," "partially hydrogenated," "hardened," and "partially hardened" mean nothing unless the type of oil is spelled out. Regardless of the fancy terms, to be on the safe side, when you want polyunsaturated oils, make sure the label reads corn, safflower, cottonseed, or soybean oil, apart from how it's processed and whether you want cooking oil or margarine.

Choosing a polyunsaturated fat or oil doesn't mean you can use all you want. Since all fats are high in calories (about 45 per teaspoon), polyunsaturated oils and fats included, they must be used with a light hand. The prudent diet also calls for maintaining a desirable weight. Two to four tablespoons daily, including what is used in cooking, on salads, or with bread, are the maximum suggested by the American Heart Association.

Despite all these warnings, there are few "X-rated" foods. *X-rated* in this case means *not* for adults over 18, although these foods may be enjoyed by youngsters, depending on their family history of stroke and heart disease. The list of X-rated foods is topped by all organ meats, including liver, shellfish, and prepared meats, such as sausage and luncheon meats, that may contain organ meats.

How to Eat Well

Still and all, no one is going to starve following the prudent diet. There is enough variety to make menu planning—and eating—enjoyable. As a matter of fact, for a look at what you can eat daily on the diet, look at this menu guide.

BREAKFAST

High vitamin C fruit or juice
High quality protein food—cottage cheese,
fish, nonfat milk
Bread—wholegrain or enriched, or cereal
Beverage

LUNCH

High quality protein food—fish, cottage cheese, poultry,
lean meat
Vegetables—cooked or raw
Bread—wholegrain or enriched
Fruit
Beverage

AFTERNOON

Snack Foods—see list

DINNER

Fruit or consommé
High quality protein food—fish, cottage cheese, poultry,
lean meat
Cooked vegetables—high vitamin A at least 4 or 5 times
per week
Raw vegetable salad with oil dressing
Potato or other starchy vegetable if you like
Bread—wholegrain or enriched if you like
Dessert—if you like: fruit or fruit gelatin, pudding, cake or
cookies made with polyunsaturated oil
Beverage

EVENING

Snack foods—see list following

SNACK FOODS

High Nutritive Value	Low Nutritive Value
Fruits and vegetables	Gelatin dessert
Nonfat milk	Water ices
Enriched or wholegrain bread and cereals	Sherbet
	Candy, hard
Nuts	Angel food cake
Cottage and pot cheese	Sponge cake
	Liquor, wine, beer

A Last Word on Cholesterol

It used to be that we considered up to 300 milligrams
of blood cholesterol safe. We think we know better

now. A safe blood cholesterol level is thought to be 180 to 200 milligrams. In any case, we think it prudent to follow a prudent diet. For different types of high blood fat disorders, additional treatment may be required.

On the average, Americans consume from 600 to 1,500 milligrams of cholesterol each day. A person who has a family history of heart disease or an elevation of blood fats should limit consumption to 300 milligrams. Considering that every 500 milligrams can raise an individual's blood cholesterol about 25 to 30 points, it doesn't take much imagination to guess what happens when cholesterol-rich foods are eaten.

Each egg yolk contains about 250 milligrams of cholesterol.

A 3-ounce serving of meat—including poultry and fish—contains from 54 to 81 milligrams. That may not sound like much in comparison to egg yolk, but remember it is the saturated fat in *beef, lamb, and pork* and their products that act in concert with cholesterol to raise the concentration level of cholesterol in the bloodstream. Poultry and fish don't contain that amount of saturated fat.

An ounce of butter contains 71 milligrams of cholesterol.

A 3-ounce serving of organ meats—liver, kidney, heart, sweetbreads—has from 375 milligrams of cholesterol to as much as 2,000 milligrams.

Crab, shrimp, and clams have twice as much cholesterol as a 3-ounce serving of lean red meat. Oysters, scallops, lobster, and caviar are so high that they, like organ meats, should be eaten sparingly, if at all, by high-risk patients.

Now for some comparisons:

The standard American breakfast of orange juice, one or two eggs fried in butter, a choice of bacon or ham or sausage, two pieces of toast with butter, and coffee with cream and sugar contains about 755 milligrams of cholesterol and 45 grams of saturated fat.

A breakfast that satisfies nutritional requirements and tastes just as good might consist of orange juice, scrambled eggs (made with egg whites only or *Egg Beaters),* a slice of whole-wheat toast with polyunsaturated margarine, and a cup of skim milk. It contains only *5 to 7* milligrams of cholesterol and 2 grams of saturated fat.

If you have a sweet tooth, listen to this. A chocolate cake made with standard ingredients contains 955 milligrams of cholesterol. One baked with cocoa and polyunsaturated fats has no cholesterol at all—and you can't tell the difference in taste! It may sound technical, but it tastes good.

Food doesn't have to taste "bad" to be "good" for you. Remember, however, that too much "good" food can be bad for you.

Good and Good for You

Cooking on a low-cholesterol, polyunsaturated-fat diet can be fun, and there is far more variety than you may realize. For example, you don't have to give up cream sauces or whipped cream—you just have to make them differently, with different ingredients. Low-cholesterol cookbooks are available, offering a full-range of all types of recipes, even gourmet. Reading all the books isn't necessary to eating sensibly, however.

As a start, here are some general cooking tips that you'll also want to keep in mind:

1. Try experimenting with lemon juice and spices on vegetables and meats, especially to keep your salt intake down. Spices, such as rosemary and dill, add a flavor all their own when cooked with vegetables or used to broil fish or chicken. Other spices that add gourmet touches are garlic, bay leaf, oregano, and celery seed. Fresh parsley and mint in season are delicious with vegetables, as are chives or the green tops of scallions. All of these spices can also be used in salad dressings and sauces.

2. If you're a sour-cream fancier, substitute yogurt instead. A low-fat yogurt with a dash of chives tops a baked potato superbly, and it can do everything in a sauce that sour cream will do. It can even be used in-stead of mayonnaise for potato or macaroni salad or cole slaw, with the addition of a dash of polyunsat-urated salad oil and vinegar and spices. You can't tell the difference!

3. If you're a whipped-cream fancier, you can still enjoy whipped "cream" although you stay away from prepared whipped toppings (often made with coconut oil) that may be high in cholesterol and/or saturated fat. The labels on evaporated or powdered skim milk often give instructions on whipping, and we have in-cluded one recipe in this chapter.

4. Whenever you cook meat, trim off all the fat. If you're stewing or cooking with liquids, you can always let the dish cool until the fat comes to the surface and is more easily skimmed off. Reheating often improves the flavor of these dishes, too.

So please don't say, "There is 'nothing' to eat on a low-cholesterol diet." There's plenty, and these tips will help you enjoy your meals. Just to give you an idea of how well you can eat on what, at this point, may seem an X-rated diet, here are a few recipes for you to try. Remember, every time oil is mentioned—even if it isn't said or specified—be sure to use a polyunsaturated oil, preferably corn, safflower, or walnut oil. (Recipes marked with one asterisk (*) are from the New York City *Prudent Diet;* those marked with two asterisks (**), are from *Cooking with Fleischmann's Egg Beaters.)*

SALAD DRESSINGS

French Dressing*

1 cup oil	*1 teaspoon sugar*
¼ cup cider vinegar	*1 teaspoon salt*

Lemon juice may be substituted for all or part of vinegar. Measure all ingredients into a bottle or jar. Cover tightly and shake well. Chill several hours. Shake thoroughly before serving. For variation, add any or all of the following: ½ teaspoon paprika, dry mustard, 1 clove garlic. Garlic should be removed before dressing is stored.

Use French Dressing for raw salad greens, cooked string beans, asparagus, broccoli; marinating and basting meat and fish.

Variations of French Dressing*

Herb Dressing: To 1 cup of French Dressing add 1 teaspoon dried herbs or 1 tablespoon fresh herbs. Use for sliced tomatoes, raw salad greens. Examples of herbs are tarragon, chervil, chives, dill, sweet basil and oregano. Use your favorites and experiment with others.

Red Oil Dressing: To 1 cup of French Dressing add ⅔ cup catsup and 1 clove garlic. Use for tossed green salad, on avocado with grapefruit sections.

Mock Sour Cream*

2 tablespoons lemon juice
3 tablespoons nonfat liquid milk or buttermilk
8 oz. cottage cheese
chopped chives, optional

Put lemon juice and milk in blender. Add cottage cheese gradually while on low speed. Blend 2 to 5 minutes on high speed. If, on standing, cream becomes too thick,

thin it out with nonfat liquid milk or buttermilk to desired consistency. Add chives if desired. Mix well.

Cottage Cheese Salad Dressing*

8 oz. cottage cheese
¼ cup cider vinegar
¾ cup buttermilk
1 teaspoon oregano

½ teaspoon garlic powder
1 teaspoon salt
1 teaspoon sugar
2 stalks scallions, chopped
   finely

Whip the cottage cheese in a blender until it becomes
liquid. Remove and place in a bowl. Add remaining
ingredients and mix well. Chill before serving. Use Cottage Cheese Salad Dressing for fruit, vegetable, and
seafood salads.

Yogart (Fat-free)*

For this yogurt, less water is used (in proportion to nonfat dry milk) than when making nonfat liquid milk.
This produces a more concentrated product.

1 cup notfat milk (enough to make 1 quart of nonfat
   liquid milk)
3 cups water only
¼ cup plain yogurt

Mix nonfat dry milk and water. Slowly bring to a boil.
Cool to luke warm temperature. Thin out yogurt by adding ½ cup of the lukewarm milk. Stir well to make it
smooth. Add yogurt mixture to the rest of milk and
blend thoroughly. Pour into serving-size cups. Cover
them with thick towel. Paper toweling between cups
helps maintain even, warm temperature. Leave undis-
turbed for about 5 to 6 hours, free from drafts and jolts.
Refrigerate after it solidifies. Save some yogurt to start
a new batch.

For variety: Add fresh or stewed fruit, berries or spices.

SOUP

New England Fish Chowder*

1 cup water	*2 tablespoons oil*
½ teaspoon salt	*¼ cup chopped onion*
dash of pepper	*1½ cups diced raw*
1 lb. fish—cod, haddock,	*potatoes*
whiting or halibut	*1 cup warmed nonfat*
	liquid milk
	chopped parsley or paprika

Boil water. Add salt, pepper and fish. Simmer 15-20 minutes (do not boil). Remove bones and skin. Flake the fish. Strain the stock. In a pot, heat oil and add onion. Cook until transparent. Add fish stock and potatoes to the onion. Boil 15 minutes until potatoes are done. Add milk and flaked fish. Simmer 2-3 minutes. Let stand a few minutes to blend flavors. Garnish with chopped parsley or paprika. Serves 3.

SAUCES

White Sauce*

2 tablespoons oil	*1 cup nonfat liquid milk*
2 tablespoons flour	*salt and pepper to taste*

Heat oil. Add flour; cook while stirring. Have heat low enough so that flour mixture remains light in color. Stir the milk in slowly. Bring to a boil and cook for a few minutes. Season with salt and pepper. Makes 1 cup.

Broth or vegetable or fish stock may be used for all or part of milk, depending upon the kind of food the sauce is to be served with. Vary the flavor of the white sauce by adding any one of the following—celery salt, onion juice, lemon juice, grated nutmeg, Worcestershire sauce, chopped chives, dill, parsley.

Serve white sauce with vegetables such as broccoli, asparagus, cauliflower, carrots or fish and poultry.

Curry Sauce*

¼ cup onion chopped
4 tablespoons oil
½ to 1 teaspoon curry
powder
1 medium peeled, chopped
tart apple

2½ tablespoons flour
1 cup broth (chicken, beef,
shrimp or vegetable)
1 cup nonfat liquid milk
1 tablespoon lemon juice
salt to taste

Sauté onion in oil until tender. Add curry powder, apple and continue cooking for about 10 minutes over low heat. Stir in flour and blend until smooth. Slowly add broth, then milk, bring to a boil. Cook for 5 minutes. Add lemon juice and salt to taste. Serve with fish, leftover veal or chicken, over boiled rice. Yields 2 cups.

BREAKFAST AND LUNCH DISHES

Puffy Omelet**

1 cup (1 container) Fleischmann's Egg Beaters
¼ teaspoon salt
1/16 teaspoon cream of tartar
2 teaspoons corn oil

Combine Egg Beaters, salt and cream of tartar in small mixer bowl. Beat on high speed of electric mixer for 5 minutes. Heat corn oil in a heavy 8-inch skillet over low heat, tilting pan to coat with oil. Pour in beaten Egg Beaters. Heat without stirring for 5 minutes, or until bottom is set. Place skillet in preheated 325° F. oven for 5 minutes. Loosen edges of omelet with spatula. Fold in half. Lift out onto serving plate. Serve with desired sauce. Serves 2.

Tomato Sauce: Melt 3 tablespoons margarine in skillet. Add 1½ cups peeled, seeded, coarsely chopped fresh tomatoes, 1 clove crushed garlic, 1 teaspoon chopped chives, ¼ teaspoon salt, ⅛ teaspoon basil leaves and a dash of pepper. Bring mixture to a boil. Reduce heat; simmer 10 minutes, stirring occasionally. If desired, thicken with 1 teaspoon flour.

Mushroom Sauce: Sauté ¼ pound sliced mushrooms in 2 tablespoons margarine. Blend in 1 tablespoon flour, ⅛ teaspoon salt and ¼ teaspoon beef flavor base. Add ½ cup water and ½ teaspoon Worcestershire sauce. Cook and stir until mixture comes to a boil.

Honey Lemon Sauce: Combine 2 tablespoons hot melted margarine, 2 tablespoons honey, 2 teaspoons lemon juice and ⅛ teaspoon salt.

French Toast**

1 cup (1 container) Fleischmann's Egg Beaters
⅛ teaspoon salt
6 slices white bread (day-old)
2 tablespoons Fleischmann's margarine
Table syrup, confectioners' sugar or jelly

Combine Egg Beaters and salt in a shallow dish and use to coat bread on both sides. Fry in margarine over medium-low heat until golden brown on both sides. Serve hot with table syrup, confectioners' sugar or jelly. Makes 3 servings.

Pancakes**

2 cups unsifted flour
3 teaspoons baking powder
2 teaspoons sugar
1 teaspoon salt
1¾ cups skim milk
½ cup (½ container) Fleischmann's Egg Beaters
¼ cup corn oil
Fleischmann's margarine
Pancake syrup

In a mixing bowl blend together flour, baking powder, sugar and salt. Combine milk, Egg Beaters and corn oil. Add to dry ingredients. Beat with rotary beater just until mixture is well blended and only a few small lumps remain.

For each pancake, pour ¼ cup batter onto a hot, lightly oiled griddle. Cook until pancakes are bubbly and edges look dry. Turn and cook until browned on underside. Serve with margarine and syrup. Makes 4 servings (12 to 14 pancakes).

Waffles: Pour batter into hot waffle iron to spread to 1-inch from edge. Bake until steaming stops. Makes 4 servings (14 4-inch waffles).

MEAT DISHES

Braised Chicken—Chinese Style*

1 frying chicken, cut into serving-size pieces	½ lb. mushroom caps
1 clove garlic, crushed	2 tablespoons sherry
2 tablespoons vegetable oil	2 tablespoons soy sauce

Brown chicken and garlic lightly in oil. Add soy sauce and sherry, and cook for 3 minutes. Add mushrooms, cover and simmer until tender (about 20-30 minutes). Serves 4.

Oven-Fried Chicken*

¼ cup lemon juice	¼ teaspoon powdered thyme
¼ cup oil	
½ teaspoon salt	1 frying chicken, cut into serving-size pieces
⅛ teaspoon pepper	

Combine lemon juice, oil and seasoning to make a marinade. Pour over chicken parts. Be sure the chicken parts are well covered with marinade. Let stand at least one hour in refrigerator. Bake in moderate oven 350° skin side down for about 25-30 minutes. Turn chicken, skin side up for 25-30 minutes. Serves 4.

Chicken Paprika*

2 medium-size onions,
  sliced
3 tablespoons oil
2-3 teaspoons paprika
1 frying chicken, disjointed

salt and pepper
1 tablespoon flour
⅓ cup chicken broth or
  water
1 teaspoon lemon juice or
  1 tablespoon white wine

Preheat oven to 325°. Sauté onions in oil until golden. Add paprika and mix. Add chicken pieces, tossing them around until well coated with the onion. Sprinkle with salt and pepper. Cover and bake about 45 minutes. Remove chicken pieces. Keep warm. Mix flour with chicken broth or water and add to pan juices. Add lemon juice or wine. Cook for a few minutes. Pour over chicken. Serve with rice or noodles. Serves 4.

Baked Fish*

2 medium-size onions
4 tablespoons oil
1 No. 2 can tomatoes
1 clove garlic, crushed
½ teaspoon paprika
1 teaspoon salt

juice of ½ lemon
2 lbs fish (striped bass, red
  snapper, carp, mackerel,
  or other fish)
chopped parsley
lemon slices

Cut onion into thin slices and sauté in 2 tablespoons oil until golden. Add tomatoes, garlic, paprika, salt, lemon juice and remaining oil. Simmer about 20 minutes. Place fish in baking dish and cover with sauce. Bake in preheated oven at 350°, approximately 30 minutes. Before serving, garnish with chopped parsley and lemon slices. Serves 4.

Salmon Steak Baked in Wine*

1 lb. fresh salmon slices	*juice of ½ lemon*
½ inch thick	*1 clove garlic, peeled and*
salt and pepper	*sliced (optional)*
⅓ cup dry white wine or	*2 tablespoons oil*
dry sherry	

Preheat oven to 400°. Sprinkle salmon slices with salt and pepper on all sides. Place salmon slices in baking pan. Combine remaining ingredients and pour over fish. Bake about 15-20 minutes or until fish flakes easily when tested with a fork. This fish may be served hot or cold. Serves 3.

The same method of preparation may be used for many kinds of fish steaks, and also for whole fish, such as white fish or striped bass, adjusting cooking time to weight and thickness of fish.

Note: Fish flesh is naturally tender. It is cooked to develop flavor, not to make it tender. It will toughen and shrink if the fish is overcooked. Fresh fish is tastier when eaten soon after purchased.

Veal and Pepper*

3 green, 1 red medium-size	*¼ lb. mushrooms, sliced*
peppers, seeded and cut	*1 cup canned tomatoes,*
into 1-inch strips	*drained and slightly*
4 tablespoons oil	*broken up with a fork*
1 lb. boneless veal (rump,	*(or tomato purée)*
shoulder or leg) cut into	
1½-inch pieces	

Sauté peppers in 2 tablespoons oil until brown or black spots develop. This contributes to the good flavor of the dish. Remove peppers from pan. In the same pan brown veal cubes in the remaining oil. Add mushrooms and cook for about 10 minutes. Place the veal mixture in baking dish. Add tomatoes, peppers and seasoning. Cover and bake about 1 hour in 325° oven. Serves 3-4.

Veal Goulash*

1 lb. boneless veal	1 tablespoon oil
3 tablespoons flour	¾ cup thinly sliced onions
½ teaspoon salt	1 teaspoon paprika
dash of pepper	4 oz. tomato sauce

Trim all visible fat from the meat and cut into 1-inch cubes. Dip veal into a mixture of flour, salt, and pepper. Heat oil in a Dutch oven. Sauté onions about 10 minutes. Sprinkle with paprika. Add the meat and brown well on all sides. Add tomato sauce. Cover and cook over low heat 1 hour or until tender. Serves 4.

London Broil*

2 to 2½ lbs. flank or rump   2 tablespoons soy sauce
   of beef

Rub meat with soy sauce on both sides. Let stand 1 to 2 hours. Broil in preheated broiler to desired doneness. Slice thin. Serves 8. A tender, juicy, flavorful steak from a lean cut of beef.

Meat Loaf**

3 pounds lean ground beef	1 large garlic clove
2 cups fresh bread crumbs	½ cup (½ container)
½ cup chopped onion	Fleischmann's Egg
¼ cup chopped green	Beaters
pepper	½ cup catsup
¼ cup minced parsley	⅓ cup water
1 tablespoon salt	2 tablespoons
½ teaspoon oregano	Worcestershire sauce
leaves	

In large bowl combine all ingredients. Press mixture into an ungreased loaf pan (9″ x 5″ x 3″). Bake at 350° F. 1½ hours. Drain off excess fat. Invert loaf onto serving dish. Let stand several minutes before slicing. Makes 12 servings.

Breaded Veal Cutlets**

1 teaspoon salt
½ teaspoon paprika
1 pound thin veal cutlets
  (4 pieces)
1 cup fine dry bread
  crumbs

1 tablespoon minced
  parsley
½ cup (½ container)
  Fleischmann's Egg
  Beaters
Corn oil
Lemon slices

Combine salt and paprika; sprinkle evenly over cutlets. Pound cutlets with mallet to flatten. Combine bread crumbs and parsley. Dip cutlets into Egg Beaters; then coat with bread crumb mixture. Place on wire rack to dry for 15 minutes. Fry in hot (375° F.) corn oil, ¼ inch deep, 3 to 4 minutes on each side, or until done. Drain on paper towels. Garnish with lemon slices. Makes 4 servings.

BREADS

Muffins**

2 cups unsifted flour
⅓ cup sugar
3 teaspoons baking powder
¾ teaspoon salt
¼ cup (½ stick) Fleisch-
  mann's margarine

1 cup skim milk
½ cup (½ container)
  Fleischmann's Egg
  Beaters

Mix flour, sugar, baking powder and salt. Cut in margarine until pieces are size of small peas. Combine skim milk and Egg Beaters. Add to flour mixture. Stir quickly with fork just until dry ingredients are moistened. (Batter will be lumpy.) Divide mixture evenly among 12 greased muffin pans, 2¾" x 1¼". Bake at 400° F. 25 minutes, or until done. Serve hot. Yields 12.

Blueberry Muffins: Add 1 cup fresh blueberries, washed, drained and dried, with milk mixture.

Bran Muffins: Substitute 1½ cups whole-bran cereal for 1 cup of flour.

Corn Bread**

1 cup yellow corn meal
1 cup unsifted flour
2 tablespoons sugar
4 teaspoons baking powder
½ teaspoon salt

⅓ cup Fleischmann's margarine
1 cup skim milk
½ cup (½ container) Fleischmann's Egg Beaters

In large bowl combine corn meal, flour, sugar, baking powder and salt. Cut in margarine. Blend together milk and Egg Beaters. Stir into corn meal mixture. Beat for one minute. Pour into greased 8-inch square baking dish. Bake at 425° F. 20 to 25 minutes, or until done. Makes 9 servings.

Corn Muffins: Pour batter into 12 greased 3" x 1½" muffin pans. Bake at 400° F. 20 to 25 minutes.

Corn Sticks: Pour batter into 24 well-greased corn stick pans, filling each about ⅔ full. Bake at 425° F. 15 to 20 minutes.

Spoon Bread**

½ cup white corn meal	⅔ cup skim milk
1 teaspoon sugar	⅓ cup Fleischmann's Egg
½ teaspoon salt	Beaters
¾ cup boiling water	2 teaspoons baking powder
¼ cup (½ stick) Fleisch-	Fleischmann's margarine
mann's margarine	

Combine corn meal, sugar, and salt in mixing bowl. Gradually stir in boiling water. Add margarine; break up and stir until melted. Allow to cool. Stir in milk and Egg Beaters, then blend in baking powder. Pour into an ungreased 1-quart casserole. Bake at 325° F. for 30 to 35 minutes, or until a silver knife inserted in center comes out clean. Serve hot with Fleischmann's margarine.

DESSERTS

Apple Cake**

1⅓ cups unsifted flour	½ cup (½ container)
2½ teaspoons baking	Fleischmann's Egg
powder	Beaters
¼ teaspoon salt	½ teaspoon vanilla extract
¾ cup sugar	½ cup skim milk
1 teaspoon ground	½ cup dark seedless
cinnamon	raisins
⅓ cup softened Fleisch-	4 cups sliced pared apples
mann's margarine	

Combine flour, baking powder, and salt. Stir to blend; set aside. Blend together ¼ cup sugar and cinnamon; set aside. In small mixer bowl cream margarine and remaining ½ cup sugar until light. Beat in Egg Beaters and vanilla extract. Beating on low speed, alternately add flour mixture and milk, beginning and ending with dry ingredients. Fold in raisins. Turn batter into a greased 8-inch square baking pan. Arrange apple slices on batter in rows. Sprinkle with cinnamon-sugar. Bake at 375° F. about 1 hour, or until done. Cool cake in pan. Best when served warm. Makes 9 servings.

Pecan Sticky Buns**

3 to 4 cups unsifted flour
¼ cup sugar
1 teaspoon salt
1 package active dry yeast
½ cup skim milk
¼ cup water
⅓ cup Fleischmann's margarine

½ cup (½ container) Fleischmann's Egg Beaters (at room temperature)
¼ cup (½ stick) Fleischmann's margarine, melted
½ cup firmly packed dark brown sugar

Mix 1 cup flour, sugar, salt, and yeast. Combine milk, water, and ⅓ cup margarine. Heat over low heat until very warm (120° F.–130° F.). Gradually add to dry ingredients; beat 2 minutes at medium speed, scraping bowl occasionally. Add Egg Beaters and ½ cup flour. Beat at high speed for 2 minutes. Stir in additional flour to make a soft dough. Turn onto lightly floured board; knead until smooth and elastic (8 to 10 minutes). Place in greased bowl, turn to grease top. Cover; let rise in warm place, free from draft, until doubled in bulk, about 1 hour. Meanwhile, prepare pans. Punch dough down; divide in half. Roll each to a 14″ x 9″ rectangle. Brush with melted margarine; sprinkle with brown sugar. Roll up to form rolls, 9 inches long. Pinch seams to seal. Cut each into 1-inch slices. Arrange cut side up in pans. Cover; let rise until doubled, about 45 minutes. Bake at 375° F. for 20 to 25 minutes, or until done. Cool 10 minutes in pans. Invert rolls onto plates to cool. Makes 18 rolls.

To prepare pans: Melt ½ cup margarine. Stir in 1 cup firmly packed dark brown sugar and ½ cup light corn syrup. Heat and stir until sugar is dissolved. Pour into 2 greased 8-inch square baking pans. Sprinkle each with ½ cup pecan pieces.

Flaky Pastry*

2 cups sifted flour
¼ teaspoon cinnamon
(optional)
1 teaspoon salt

½ cup oil
5 tablespoons cold skim
milk or water

Sift together flour, cinnamon, and salt. Combine oil and milk in measuring cup. Beat with a fork until thickened and creamy. To avoid separation, immediately pour all at once over the flour mixture. Toss and mix with a fork. The dough will be moist. Form into ball and divide in half. Shape each half into a flat round. Roll between two 12-inch squares of wax paper (paper will not slip if table is wiped with damp cloth). Roll out until dough forms circle, reaching edges of paper. Remove top sheet of wax paper. Invert dough over pie pan. Peel off the other paper. Fit pastry into pan and trim edges. Roll out top crust in the same way. Cut gashes for steam to escape. Fill pastry-lined pan with desired filling. Place top crust over filling and trim ½ inch beyond rim of pan. Seal edge by folding top crust under bottom crust. Flute edge. Bake at 400° for 15 minutes, reduce heat to 350° and continue baking for 30 to 45 minutes until done. Use with any pie filling. Yields one 2-crust 8- or 9-inch pie. For a one-crust pie, make one-half of the recipe. Roll out as above and fit into pie pan. Prick surface of crust. Bake at 450° for 10 to 12 minutes.

How to Whip Evaporated Milk*

Pour milk (undiluted) into freezer tray or directly into bowl for whipping. Chill in freezer compartment until fine crystals begin to form around the edges. Pour into cold bowl and whip rapidly with cold beater until very stiff. When properly handled, it will whip as stiff as cream. If milk does not whip well, it is not cold enough. Just rechill and whip again.

Southern Pecan Pie**

¼ cup (½ stick) Fleisch-
   mann's margarine
1 cup sugar
¾ cup light corn syrup
¾ cup (¾ container)
   Fleischmann's Egg
   Beaters

1 teaspoon vanilla extract
1¾ cups pecans
1 unbaked 9-inch pastry
   shell

Melt margarine over low heat. Remove from heat; mix in sugar and corn syrup. Blend in Egg Beaters and vanilla extract. Add pecans. Pour into pie shell. Bake at 350° F. for 35 to 40 minutes, or until done. Makes one 9-inch pie.

Maple Walnut Pie: Proceed as above, except substitute ½ teaspoon maple flavoring for vanilla extract and walnuts for pecans.

Rice Custard**

1½ cups skim milk
⅓ cup sugar
¼ teaspoon salt
2 tablespoons Fleisch-
   mann's margarine

1 cup (1 container)
   Fleischmann's Egg
   Beaters
1 cup cooked rice
½ cup dark seedless
   raisins
1 teaspoon vanilla extract

Scald milk; add sugar, salt, and margarine. Stir until margarine is melted. Add milk mixture slowly to Egg Beaters, stirring constantly. Stir in rice, raisins and vanilla extract. Divide mixture evenly among seven 6-ounce custard cups. Set in a pan of hot water about 1 inch deep. Bake at 350° F. 30 minutes, or until knife inserted in center of custard comes out clean. Makes 7 servings.

Spicy Rice Custard: Proceed as above but stir in ¼ teaspoon ground nutmeg with vanilla extract.

Bread Pudding**

2 cups skim milk	*1 teaspoon vanilla extract*
½ cup sugar	*½ teaspoon ground*
½ cup (½ container)	*cinnamon*
Fleischmann's Egg	*¼ teaspoon salt*
Beaters	*2 cups 1-inch bread cubes*

Combine milk, sugar, Egg Beaters, vanilla extract, cinnamon, and salt in a large bowl. Stir in bread cubes. Divide mixture evenly among five 6-ounce custard cups. Set in a pan of hot water about 1 inch deep. Bake at 350° F. for 40 minutes, or until knife inserted in center of custard comes out clean. Makes 5 servings.

Raisin Bread Pudding: Proceed as above but substitute ⅓ cup dark seedless raisins for ¼ cup sugar.

Chapter XI

HOW TO STOP SMOKING

Smoking is a definite risk factor in the causing of heart disease and cancer of the lung. The evidence is convincing. The statistics are confirmatory. Although the connection to stroke is also clear, because of the many health hazards, our attention should be devoted to the *prevention* of smoking.

The best and simplest way to stop smoking is never to start smoking in the first place. So, if you haven't started, don't begin now. If you have started to smoke, stop. It's never too late—or is it?

Since there is evidence that the younger you start smoking, the more you smoke, and the longer you go on smoking, there is every reason for parents to discourage their children from smoking. Unfortunately, children learn by example more than by lecture, so if parents smoke, all the talk and the good reasons for not starting may have a negative rather than a positive effect on children. Conversely, children should be a good enough reason for parents to stop smoking.

How to stop smoking, then, actually involves two factors: How *not* to start in the first place and how to stop if you already smoke. Assuming that a person who hasn't started to smoke probably won't begin to smoke once he—or she—reaches his twenties, the emphasis here is on reaching teen-agers (who may or may not smoke) and adults who smoke cigarettes.

Youngsters and Cigarettes

When we say teen-agers, we mean boys *and* girls. Although both strokes and heart attacks claim more men than women, we don't know whether it is because the male sex is more prone to cardiovascular disease than women or because environmental factors predispose the male of the species more to strokes and heart attacks than they do women. We do know that men have been smoking for a longer time and more heavily than women, at least until recent years. Nowadays, however, the difference between the sexes is narrowing. Perhaps coincidental to this closing of the statistical gap is the fact that more women smoke and smoke more heavily than they used to. We know, too, that women who are heavy smokers have smaller babies, run a higher risk of miscarriage, and take a greater chance of losing their babies in the first year of life.

The emphasis *not* to smoke, then, should be equal, without distinction as to sex, although some arguments may be more effective with boys than with girls—or with girls rather than boys. Male and female peer groups behave and respond differently.

Parents will know which reasons will or should work best with their children, but here is a rundown of some arguments to use to convince youngsters not to smoke. What must be kept in mind is that teen-agers often "try out" smoking as they do alcohol—out of curiosity, to be a big shot, to appear sophisticated, *or to satisfy their peer group.*

Forbidden fruits are often sweeter. Adults, if they're honest with themselves, can remember how they felt in their teens and what their reactions were to being simply forbidden to do something and how they felt about smoking or drinking or both. Recalling these feelings may help them reach their own children. The important thing is that just to forbid a child to smoke may not be enough, unless you can offer reasons appealing to logic and the discipline that may be needed to enforce what you say.

Discipline may infringe on peer-group expectations. Peer-group behavior is difficult to penetrate. It has its own secrecy, loyalty, and *esprit de corps.* If not *motivated properly,* the peer group can be self-destructive (for example, smoking, drug abuse). Athletically motivated groups and social groups organized around a purpose (4-H, a Y, and so on) usually have no problems with smoking. What peer groups could use is leadership by *nonrelated* adults who are sympathetic to the serious problems of adolescence. Peer rewards for not smoking should be encouraged.

And now for some "logical" reasons to use with your youngsters.

Health. Telling a child that smoking is a path to lung disease, cancer, heart attacks, and strokes will probably have little effect in the teens, unless the youngster has a close relative, or knows someone he or she admires, who had one of these diseases. Boys who are athletically inclined will react more favorably to the effects of cigarettes on their playing abilities. Smoking does cut down their lung capacity, which in turn affects their ability to run as far and as fast or to swim, not to mention their overall stamina. Holding up a nonsmoking athlete whom the youngster admires may help. Our athletes could and should do more in this regard.

Girls are less inclined to be as athletic. If they are, the same arguments may sway them. A teen-age star like tennis player Chris Evert, who is attractive, popular, and successful, is a good example. A girl may be more swayed by the next argument.

Weight control. Teen-agers have probably heard their elders say all too often, "If I gave up smoking, I'd gain weight," "I tried to stop smoking, and I started to gain weight," or similar statements. The fact is, smoking will *not* help anyone to lose weight. There is only one way to lose weight, and that's by reducing calorie intake. If a youngster is sincere about losing weight, the family physician can offer helpful recommendations, after making sure that the youngster has no physical reasons for being overweight and really needs to lose weight in the first place.

Sophistication. You don't have to smoke to be "smart," and it's smarter not to smoke. A youngster who feels awkward in social situations can be helped to feel more at ease with a little help and attention. These years are an awkward age for many teenagers. Encouraging a youngster's interests and helping the teen-ager to feel at ease may prevent his starting to smoke and putting on an act of being at ease. If the youngster is copying someone he feels is "sophisticated," you can point to many public figures, including movie stars who have given up smoking (for example, John Wayne, Gene Kelly, Arthur Godfrey).

Stop smoking, if you yourself smoke. Children copy their elders. You can best encourage a youngster by showing that you know smoking is harmful. You might also try to invite friends who don't smoke to your house or ask smoking friends not to smoke when the youngsters are around. If youngsters see *you* can have fun without smoking, they may not start.

Expense. Smoking is an expensive habit. Pointing out to a youngster that money spent on cigarettes could be spent on other, more enjoyable pastimes may be a form of bribery, but a youngster on an allowance probably has more ways of *spending* money than—money! Explaining what a pack of cigarettes costs and how the money can be used in other ways is an economic fact of life that may not only convince the youngster for the moment but also keep the child convinced later on.

Three packs of cigarettes may be the equivalent of a movie or ball-game ticket, for example. A carton may be the price of a new pair of jeans. If a parent uses a little imagination and knows what the youngster likes, this can be a very convincing argument.

There are many other reasons for a youngster not to start smoking, many individual to the child. Not every reason will work with every teen-ager, but any reason or all reasons a parent can find are reason enough, providing they work. As the saying goes, it's a wise parent who knows his own child!

One other point: If, after talking and discussing why a youngster shouldn't smoke, you find a pack of cigarettes in a boy or girl's pocket, *don't panic!*

Losing your temper and shouting won't help, even if it does make you feel better. Sit down and talk to the youngster again and try to find out his or her *own* reasons for smoking. It may be a one-time experiment or the youngster may be "holding the pack for a friend," but it's up to you to find out. You can't expect that one talk with a youngster will be enough—keeping a child from smoking is a long-term educational project that requires discipline and understanding on your part. That discipline may mean you have to stop smoking.

The one argument you cannot answer is, "But *you* smoke!"

How to Stop Smoking—Yourself

The only way to stop smoking is to do just that: Stop. Some people can quit "cold turkey," throw out the pack and never light another. More people, despite the best motivation in the world, can't do that. The longer and the more a person smokes, the more difficult it is to give up smoking. Even fully understanding the health reasons doesn't make stopping smoking any easier. So, what can you do and how can you stop smoking?

Assuming you *really* want to stop—and this is the

first and probably the most important step—begin by following these simple steps:

(1) *Ask yourself, "Why do I smoke?"* Habitual smokers generally smoke for one or a combination of reasons. According to them:

They're nervous and they use cigarettes to hide anger, fear, frustration, inadequacy in certain situations, and so on. Cigarettes give them "something to do," especially with their hands.

They've formed a habit and often don't even know when they're smoking so they don't even really enjoy it.

They use cigarettes as a "stimulant," to wake up in the morning or get themselves going, despite the fact that cigarettes are actually a long-term depressant.

They use them as a form of pleasure, with a drink, coffee after meals, coffee breaks during the day, and in many other ways.

They're real "addicts" with a physical craving that demands more and more cigarettes to satisfy.

2. *Make out a list of the reasons why you smoke.* Then make out a list of the reasons why you shouldn't smoke. If you can't think of any reasons, look at Part I especially Chapter VII, again. Don't try to do it in your head—put the reasons on paper so you can study them and add to them, if need be. See which list is more "reasonable" and longer, and keep both handy so you can refer to them any time your motivation flags.

3. *Make out a plan of action.* Only you can decide what will work for you, but write out what you decide, so you can refer to this, too, and try to get a friend (who doesn't smoke) to help and encourage you.

All three steps are effective, whether you quit cold turkey (immediate cessation) or gradually. In both instances, success seems to depend on a few "simple" rules:

Think "now"—each day, hour, and minute is a new start. If you want a cigarette, put off the decision.

If you travel, avoid smoking compartments on trains or planes.

If you're meeting someone, pick a place where you won't be tempted to smoke if you're early or the other person is late.

If you have a choice, choose friends to meet or visit who don't smoke, at least until you've passed the first temptation to light up.

If you smoke with or after coffee, don't drink coffee.

If you're a man, switching to a pipe or cigars is "copping out." These switchers usually go back to cigarettes.

Above all, think positive, by telling yourself that you *can* stop, that you don't have to be a slave to a habit.

Now for the first way to stop smoking. The most drastic way is to say, "This is it," and quit cold turkey. No more cigarettes means not one single cigarette. 50 percent of those smokers who stop do it this way, according to figures gathered by the American Cancer Society.

During the first few weeks or so, you may want to carry gum or hard candy as substitutes when you're away from home. Celery or carrot sticks will help at home and avoid the calories of cookies or sweets if you feel like nibbling something. You may find it easier not to start again, too, if you get rid of all reminders of smoking at home or where you work: Hide or throw out ash trays, matches, lighters, cigarette cases—anything you used when you smoked.

Changing your routine and avoiding people and activities that you associate with smoking, if possible, may make it easier for you to stop by keeping temptation away from your doorstep. When you feel like reaching for a cigarette, reach for a pencil and figure out how much money you have saved already—and what you will do with the money you're going to save. If you find yourself with time on your hands, instead of watching television or reading or doing something that reminds you of smoking, try exercising or going for a walk and see how much your stamina increases. Notice, too, how much better food tastes.

If you have tried quitting cold turkey and you "can't," there are other ways. Again, make out a list, this time of when you smoke and why. For example, you have a cigarette when you get up in the morning, not necessarily because you want it but to get you "going." Figure out exactly how many cigarettes you smoke and keep a record. What you do with the record depends on you: One way to use it is to start by eliminating the cigarettes you enjoy the least, gradually cutting down to the point where you can stop altogether. Another way is to keep a daily tally, wrapping the tally around your pack of cigarettes so that you have to "unwrap" the cigarettes every time you want one. Then write down the time and why you wanted the cigarette on the tally sheet, thus making it harder to smoke. You may even decide that you really don't want the cigarette.

There are many other ways of making it harder to smoke. You can buy cigarettes by the pack instead of the carton (this is more expensive, too, and it makes you aware of just how much money is going up in smoke). You can carry the cigarettes in a different place or put them across the room instead of beside you. You can also switch brands. All the time, however, it's important to keep telling yourself you are going to stop and to refer to the reasons why you know you should stop and why you want to stop.

The Public Health Service of the Department of Health, Education, and Welfare also has pointers to help smokers stop smoking. It suggests that you start by choosing a cigarette with less tar and nicotine, in order to reduce the risks of smoking. These figures are available from the Federal Trade Commission. If you are going to go to all the trouble of getting these figures, save time and stop smoking.

No matter which cigarette you smoke, don't smoke it all the way down. The shorter the butt, the greater the intake of tar and nicotine, since the length of a cigarette acts as a kind of filter. The result is that the first half of the cigarette contains 40 percent of the tar and nicotine, and the last half, 60 percent. Longer cigarettes aren't safer—not if you smoke them that much further down. As the Public Health Service says, those "extra puffs" may be "extra perils."

Taking fewer draws on each cigarette, then, helps you to stop smoking. Reducing your inhaling of the cigarette smoke also helps. The smoke that enters your lungs does the damage, not only in causing cancer but also heart disease. At the same time, remember that some smoke is absorbed by your body, regardless of whether you inhale or not.

Above all, smoke fewer cigarettes each day. The Public Health Service suggests having your first cigarette an hour later each day. It's a psychological trick in a way, but if you know you can have one later it's not the same thing as saying you won't have one—period.

How to Stop Smoking—With Help

If you really want to stop smoking, only *you* can do it. Think of it as a day-to-day resolution, and each day it may become easier to stop. If you can't stop by yourself, however, there are smoking clinics in practically every city of any size, run by various organizations. Your physician or your local American Cancer Society may be able to suggest one. Keep in mind that these clinics won't make it any easier to stop smoking. You still have to do the work, but they do give the would-be nonsmoker emotional support.

The clinics, in general, are based on behavior modification. Behavior modification is a new concept based on old principles. The great Russian physiologist, Pavlov (1849–1936), contributed to the knowledge of behavior by his study of the conditioned response. We all remember the experiment of a dog salivating in response to the offered meat when a bell rang. After a while, the dog would respond to the bell alone, salivating without the meat's being present. Behavioral modification depends, to some degree, on conditioning. We have an urge to smoke, for example, after a cocktail, or a large meal, or a cup of coffee or tea. We are "conditioned" to have an urge for that cigarette at that time. If we don't have a large meal, drink coffee or tea, or have a cocktail, we should be able to break the conditioned response.

We are also conditioned to smoking a particular brand of cigarette that comes in an easily identifiable package. We are upset if we cannot obtain that particular package. In reality, all cigarettes, depending on whether they are menthol or nonmenthol, filtered or nonfiltered, are quite similar—whatever package they come in. In blindfold tests, cigarettes of the same type cannot be told apart. If, by some chance, you can distinguish between the taste of brands, it merely means you have an excellent taste for poison.

Why *do* we depend on that package? The reason very probably is that we are conditioned to that package. Therefore, according to behavior modification, if we are going to stop smoking, we should switch brands very frequently to prove to ourselves that we—not the package—is the master!

There are other ways to get help to stop smoking. Hypnosis and drugs such as lobelline have been used with a small degree of success. Nothing can replace motivation. Motivation is the most important underlying factor in stopping smoking. It depends on two things: Being aware of the evils that are produced in the body by the tars, carbon monoxide, and nicotine in the smoke; and making up your mind to stop. If you're under nervous tension or stress because of a special project or a big business deal and you feel that you can't stop smoking in the middle of it, pick a date when the project will be finished. At the same time, reconditioning or other forms of behavior modification are possible, practical, and necessary for some people.

Keep in mind that once you have made up your mind to stop smoking and have decided how you are going to stop, you've taken more than a step—it's a leap forward. It won't be easy, particularly for the heavy smoker, but smoking is a habit, like an addiction. Addiction creates a physical or chemical change inside the body, making it dependent on the addictive substance. Cigarettes, while they are *habit-forming* and can cause very real harm to the body, are not addictive in the sense of any drug, including alcohol. But, because they *are* a habit, stopping smoking may bring about withdrawal symptoms.

The first 48 hours are the worst, most ex-smokers agree. But there may also be other symptoms as the body learns a new way of adjusting itself to fear, tension, stress, and the other emotions that used to "call for" a cigarette. You may feel a tightness in the chest, you may be dizzy, or perspire more than usual—all of which indicate anxiety. At the same time, if the symptoms persist or if you are uncomfortable, you should consult your physician, who will be able to help.

If you find yourself gaining weight, forget it. Remember, you can lose it later. Fairly often, the weight gain disappears once the person adjusts to not smoking. Again, your physician is the person who can offer you the best help in adjusting your weight.

CHAPTER XII

HIGH BLOOD PRESSURE
AND TREATMENT

Preventing high blood pressure may be a little like preventing the Mississippi from flooding. We know what causes the Mississippi to flood (rain), and we know some of the causes of high blood pressure. But we can't stop the rain as yet. To control the floods, we know enough about flood control to erect dams and levees. It's the same with high blood pressure.

A normal or average blood pressure in adults is considered to be around 120/80. A blood pressure reading of 140/90 is not necessarily considered abnormal; it may be elevated for any number of reasons (Chapter IV), but it is of concern to your physician. In fact, to get a person's usual blood pressure, it may have to be checked several times. It has been pointed out that some persons are hyperreactive to the blood pressure machine, and may need to get used to the machine and the surroundings in order to get a true reading.

Individual blood pressures may also vary for reasons other than tension or nervousness. The blood pressure increases with age. Gerontologists (physicians who specialize in diseases of aging) seem to be undecided about what is normal blood pressure in the elderly. This problem complicates the difficulty of knowing whether an increase is "normal" due to aging or is elevated because of high blood pressure disease. It does, however, seem that a young person's blood pressure is protection against stroke. Empirical observations suggest that people with normal blood pressure develop stroke less often than those with high blood pressure.

We do know that there are certain ways high blood pressure may be controlled. We also know that high blood pressure disease—hypertension—*can* be controlled, providing the problem is attacked with dedication and regularity.

High blood pressure is quite common, affecting about 10 percent of the population. This is one of the reasons for the mass screening being performed in cities all over the country, a kind of bringing medicine to the patient, if the patient doesn't go to the doctor. Another problem, besides detection of high blood pressure, is that people won't or don't take high blood pressure or other illnesses seriously if they feel well.

If the subject doesn't involve pain, diet, or sex, the public isn't easily interested—and this is the case with early high blood pressure. Most people have to be disabused of the idea that if you do have a headache, you do have high blood pressure. Actually, *headache is rare* in most patients with early, *bona fide* high blood pressure.

High blood pressure is what is known as a *lanthanic disease,* meaning a disease that lacks symptoms—until the disease goes wild. There are many lathanic diseases —and among them are tuberculosis, rheumatic fever, and mild diabetes. These different diseases have similar and common problems in diagnosis and follow-up because the patient doesn't feel sick. People know they have them and, if they do, they take their medicine for a while. Then they may forget, don't or won't renew a prescription, or don't go back to the doctor, all because they feel well for now.

Many hypertension clinics report that from 42 to 60 percent of their patients who know they have sustained high blood pressure don't return. The Henry Ford Clinic in Detroit began a hypertensive program in 1961. Within 11 months, it had lost 50 percent of its patients. After five years, 74 percent had dropped out, 9 percent had died, and 17 percent were still under treatment. This is, of course, not a reflection on that excellent clinic, but it is indicative of how too many people feel about high blood pressure.

Education and economic level seem to make little perceptible difference in why patients drop out. Nevertheless, younger people are more apt to drop out than older ones and blacks more than whites.

Practical problems in the causing of dropouts is the cost of medication *and* the side effects of the medication. While the children of the family certainly need costly new shoes, teeth fixed, and so on, they need parents who are being treated for high blood pressure more than parents who are neglecting their high blood pressure and flirting with heart trouble and stroke.

If the cost of treatment gets to be oppressive, there are many alternatives that can be used. Many insurance companies and labor unions and companies realize that it is less expensive to treat high blood pressure than heart disease or stroke. Therefore, they are encouraging the detection and treatment of high blood pressure. Again, high blood pressure clinics throughout the country, supported by voluntary, federal, state, or municipal funds, may take the sting out of the cost of treatment. If cost is a problem, your physician can probably guide you.

Side effects are another matter. There is hardly a medicine used that doesn't have some side effects. However, we can generally adjust medicine to lessen the side effects for maximum benefit. High blood pressure medications are not exceptions. They all have individual effects that can usually be tolerated. Fortunately, if a person can't take one type of medicine, there are others that can be used.

Treating high blood pressure is your business—and helping to prevent and helping to lower and control high blood pressure makes good sense. You, in fact, are in the driver's seat. Steering along the right course will avoid an accident—a cerebrovascular accident (stroke).

What You Can Do

There are certain general measures that can be taken by anyone with high blood pressure. In some people these measures may be sufficient in themselves to bring down the blood pressure and avoid the use of medications.

A prudent diet, such as the diet in Chapter IX, aimed at lowering blood cholesterol levels and keeping them low, is equally good for anyone with high blood pressure. There is one qualification: Keep salt at a minimum. There does seem to be a relationship between the amount of salt in the diet and high blood pressure. We aren't sure of the mechanism but we are impressed by the rampant nature of high blood pressure disease in Asiatics and blacks. Both groups use a relatively high amount of salt and have a high incidence of stroke.

Remember that most food contains hidden amounts of salt. For example, you can't see or taste the salt in milk but it's there in abundance. There are about 500 milligrams of sodium in each quart of milk.

The American black has the most severe problem of high blood pressure. The social and economic pressures on this minority group are considered by some to be a significant factor in the genesis of high blood pressure. In addition, there may be a predisposing genetic factor. Diet also seems to be implicated by virtue of a high salt intake. Pork (including salt pork and bacon), ham, and "soul food" contain large amounts of salt. Certainly it would do no harm for all of us to reduce our salt intake. As for the social and economic pressures, the struggle to reduce them must continue, however difficult it is.

In the 1940s, an effective diet for the treatment of hypertensive disease was the Kempner rice diet. Its effectiveness was considered due to a markedly reduced intake of sodium chloride (salt). Whereas the average daily intake of sodium chloride is about 8 to 10 grams (8,000 to 10,000 milligrams), the salt intake on the Kempner rice diet approximated 200 milligrams. By and large, such extremes aren't presently necessary. Still, all grossly salted foods should be eliminated. This means corned, smoked, and cured foods. In addition, no salt should be used in preparing food at mealtimes. Use other spices to taste. (See Chapter X.)

Diet is not the only factor.

Emotions (such as stress, anxiety, or excitement) can elevate blood pressure temporarily. If blood pressure is elevated over a period of time, it may become permanently elevated. Trying to avoid stress doesn't mean keeping worries or anxiety inside. It does mean relieving the stress, if it can't be avoided altogether, perhaps by talking it out. For those people with high blood pressure who are obviously tense, anxious, or restless, muscular relaxation techniques, from autosuggestion to yoga, may help. A reassessment of goals consistent with a life style relatively free of tension is worthwhile. More time to relax and enjoy life is necessary. This gives less time to worry—and worry never did much good anyway.

Exercise is effective, too, only if it can relax you. If you build up tensions while you exercise, you are probably doing yourself more harm than good. Any regular program of exercise will depend on your general physical condition. And don't think you can lose weight strictly by exercising. All you'll get will be a good appetite. But make no mistake about it—exercise is important to maintain and sustain your health.

Obesity may be directly related to sustained high blood pressure, and overweight does put a burden on the heart, which, in turn, may affect blood pressure. Anyone who is more than 10 percent heavier than standard weight tables for age or height runs a higher risk from high blood pressure that may lead to a heart attack or stroke. Hence, calorie control and weight reduction of the obese is as important as cholesterol control. As a matter of fact, the blood pressure very often responds to mere weight control.

You'll be better off, too, if you stop smoking. Every study of heart disease and stroke shows that people who do have sustained high blood pressure that is controlled.

Even if you give up steaks, sweet desserts, and cigarettes, you can still enjoy life. In fact, if you're healthy, you'll probably find a lot more life to enjoy. Enjoying life is probably one of the best ways to prevent hypertension in the beginning—and one way to keep it under control. If you're enjoying life, you aren't under *undue* tension or stress or anxiety. You'll also probably be getting an adequate amount of exercise—and you'll be at an advantage in living longer, more fruitfully, and more healthfully.

Cause and Treatment of High Blood Pressure

There are many causes of high blood pressure disease. In about 10 to 15 percent of the people with high blood pressure disease, we can identify a cause. We call this secondary hypertension, because the hypertension is secondary to kidney disease, disease of the adrenal glands, abnormal arteries, other rare causes, or any combination of these. The kind of high blood pressure disease that is most common (85 to 90 percent) is called *essential hypertension*. (There is nothing "essential" about it—we can do without it. *Essential* in this context is a medical term meaning that we don't know the cause.)

In attempting to ascertain the cause of high blood pressure, the physician will get a history of previous disorders, not only of the person himself who has high blood pressure, but of his family. In addition, he will perform a physical examination that will look for abnormalities that can be seen, felt, or heard. He will then want a laboratory evaluation of the hypertensive subject. The blood will be extensively studied, as well as the urine. He may require X-ray examinations before a definitive conclusion about the cause of the high blood pressure is reached. To assess the health of the heart, an electrocardiogram may be performed.

The foregoing constitutes what is basically called the hypertensive "work-up." Although it may entail significant expense, its worth can't be strictly measured in dollars and cents.

Once the physician has performed and evaluated the tests he deems necessary, he will be able to make a diagnosis. If a cause for the high blood pressure is found, appropriate action can be taken. Here is a case history of one man.

Mr. E. H. is a 30-year-old laborer who sought his physician's help because of shortness of breath. Upon making a physical examination, his physician found E.H.'s blood pressure elevated to 200/120, his heart enlarged, and decreased pulsation in his lower extremities. In addition, the blood pressure was lower in the lower extremities. Further laboratory and X-ray examinations confirmed the diagnosis of a rare disease called coarctation of the aorta. In this condition, there is high blood pressure in the upper extremities and a decreased pressure in the lower extremities because the main artery— the aorta—is pinched after it gives off its supply of blood to the upper extremities.

The diagram of coarctation of the aorta on page 72 shows graphically what happens. This condition is corrected by relieving the pinching through surgery. Thus, when Mr. E.H. was operated upon, the constriction was remedied. His blood pressure returned to normal, and his shortness of breath disappeared. His outlook is excellent.

Mrs. A. C. is an example of another type of hypertension in which there is a physical cause. She is a 42-year-old hypertensive woman who had attacks of nervousness, headaches, and tremulousness. The laboratory examination revealed an elevation of a hormonal by-product of adrenalin in her urine. Further studies confirmed the diagnosis of a tumor of the adrenal gland. She was operated on for this exceedingly rare condition and is perfectly well since surgery. Her blood pressure is now normal.

These are only two examples of secondary hypertension, that is, hypertension due to another cause. The point to remember is that once the *cause* is corrected, the hypertension or *high blood pressure* is corrected.

Despite these cases, let's remember that the vast majority of people with hypertension have essential hypertension (no known cause). For a long time, patients with essential hypertension weren't treated vigorously because no convincing evidence was at hand that treatment would save lives and also because adequate treatment wasn't available.

Time has changed things, on all scores. As a result of studies on high blood pressure in New Zealand and more recently in an excellently controlled Veterans Administration cooperative study, the effectiveness of drug treatment in high blood pressure seems to be convincing. One of those physicians who has devoted a professional lifetime to the study of high blood pressure is Dr. Frank Finnerty, Jr.

In the Veterans Administration cooperative study, 143 men with very high diastolic blood pressure readings of 115 milligrams of mercury or greater were divided randomly into placebo (untreated, as control) and active treatment groups. In the placebo group, there were 27 severe stroke episodes with complications; in the treated group, there were only 2 such events. There is little doubt, based on this and other studies, that the adequate treatment of high blood pressure is an important way of preventing stroke.

These studies don't mean that we have settled which of those people with high blood pressure should be treated or how they should be treated, by any means. Nevertheless, if we haven't settled the "who" or the "how," the means of treatment has improved considerably. The medical armamentarium to be used against essential hypertension has been enlarged. Still, if you are overweight, weight reduction may bring about a reduction in blood pressure without the need for medication.

The aim of medication is to reduce the blood pressure without making you miserable. This is now possible, despite the fact that virtually all medications have some side effects. Unpleasant side effects can sometimes be altered by changing the dosage, and other side effects disappear after a few weeks. For these reasons, there are a few medications worthwhile mentioning because of their widespread use and effectiveness. Since high blood pressure is epidemic, you may already be taking one of these medications. If not, one of them could one day be prescribed for you. In either case, you may want to know what the medication is all about.

Diuretics (medicine which causes the kidneys to excrete more salt in the urine) seem to potentiate—or make more effective—other medicines for lower blood pressure. There are many diuretics available for use.

The milder ones usually produce their maximum lowering effects on blood pressure in about two or three weeks. The stronger ones can bring about an increased flow of urine within hours. Diuretics are generally taken orally.

Patients taking oral diuretics are commonly encouraged to eat foods rich in potassium, since most diuretics cause not only a loss of salt but of potassium as well. Taking the diuretic in the morning with a glass of orange juice is usually quite effective. Bananas, all-bran cereals, beans, tea, and instant coffees are among foods and beverages containing ample potassium.

Exposure to high environmental temperatures causing a great deal of sweating and loss of salt through the skin in patients taking diuretics is to be avoided. If one travels to extremely warm climates, reduction in the dosage of diuretics is often called for to avoid too much salt depletion from the body. The state of heat exhaustion manifested by weakness is really the effect of not enough salt in the body. Rarely, diuretics will precipitate gout or diabetes in sensitive individuals. Such effects are controllable or generally reversible if the medication is stopped.

The brand names of some commonly used diuretics are Diuril, Lasix, and Diamox.

Reserpine is a derivative of the snake root plant, used originally in India. It has a calming effect on most people and is an effective antihypertensive (blood-pressure-lowering) medicine. It does, however, cause nasal congestion in some people and, occasionally, nightmares in others. Very rarely, it is associated with mental depression. Reserpine ordinarily takes two or three weeks to reach its full effects when taken by mouth. Its action to lower the blood pressure is increased when given with a diuretic.

Aldomet (methyldopa), another effective antihypertensive, is often accompanied by drowsiness or wooziness that usually subsides within a few weeks of use. Very rarely, an anemia may occur in sensitive individuals. Methyldopa has a greater effect than Reserpine on blood pressure. By and large, it is an effective, well-tolerated medicine.

Apresoline (hydralazine) is usually given in combination with a diuretic. A recent Veterans Administration treatment program using three drugs—Reserpine, a diuretic (hydrochlorthiazide), and hydralazine was quite effective in treating severe hypertension. Among the side effects are headaches, which generally abate as treatment proceeds. In large doses, skin rashes, joint complaints, and blood changes have been observed. These are reversed when the medication is stopped.

Ismelin (guanethidine) is a powerful blood-pressure-lowering agent, especially when used with a diuretic. Faintness or dizziness may precede falling when changes in position (from lying or sitting to standing) are performed too rapidly. It may cause diarrhea and in large doses in males, there may be sexual impotence.

It is a safe bet that the next decade will see the introduction of other medication for use in the control of high blood pressure. The aim is effectiveness, a minimum of unpleasant side effects, and last but not least, economic feasibility. Cost is a factor.

In the meantime, be sure to take the medication that your physician prescribes. Mrs. B.L. is a 38-year-old mother of five children, wife of a handyman, who decided she couldn't afford her blood-pressure medication because of the many monetary needs of her children. She refused to attend a hypertension clinic where medication was supplied free of charge, since she was too busy to wait and too proud. Mrs. B.L. had severe high blood pressure, and she suffered a right-sided stroke. Recovery was slow, but Mrs. B.L.'s blood pressure is now under good control with the faithful, daily use of medication.

If you have high blood pressure, follow your physician's advice faithfully. In fact, establish a good relationship and have trust in him. It will work both ways.

No matter how well you feel, keep taking the medication prescribed. Once high blood pressure is controlled, it still requires regular medication. Should you stop taking it, your blood pressure may stay down for a time—but it will go right back up and you'll once again be faced with the problem of getting it down and controling it.

To sum up what *you* can do about high blood pressure, here are "Ten Commandments":

1. Follow the advice of your physician.
2. Take your medication, regularly and faithfully.
3. Have periodic checkups.
4. Do not smoke.
5. Excercise according to plan.
6. Enjoy as much freedom from anxiety as possible.
7. Exercise weight control—watch your calories.
8. Stay on a prudent diet.
9. Avoid excesses of salt in your food.
10. In a positive way, enjoy life.

If these commandments are for you, your physician also has five commandments that he will follow in helping you. He will:

1. Evaluate your condition carefully.
2. Treat you with all his might and skill to get your blood pressure down and keep it down.
3. Not abandon treatment once your blood pressure comes down, because he knows that sus-

tained high blood pressure requires continuous, lifetime care.

4. Prescribe the best medication or combination of medication suited to you and to your blood pressure.

5. Follow your case as long as you both shall live!

Talking of lifetime care makes sustained high blood pressure sound expensive. It is—but its treatment is far cheaper than the cost of letting the blood pressure go untreated, resulting in heart trouble or a stroke. The goal is to prevent your having either one.

Chapter XIII

THE FUTURE AND STROKE PREVENTION

Aunt Tillie is a great old lady. She's in her 90s, drinks too much booze, eats like a horse, and smokes like a chimney. She's overweight and has had high blood pressure for forty years. She exercises by pushing herself away from the dining-room table and waddling to the television set and her favorite armchair. She says, "If I only knew that I would be 90 years old, I would have taken better care of myself!"

Aunt Tillie is the envy of everyone who knows her. She is also a medical mystery. Everyone has an Aunt Tillie—just as everyone has had an Uncle Charley. Uncle Charley had a stroke at 43.

In retrospect, why did Uncle Charley have a stroke at 43 years of age? What were the factors that Uncle Charley had that Aunt Tillie didn't have? And, by the same token, what chemistry is there in Aunt Tillie that has protected her from stroke? What environmental influences were different in Aunt Tillie and Uncle Charley?

The answers to these questions get down to the root causes of stroke and the factors that increase or decrease our chances of getting stroke. We have learned a great deal, but we have much to learn. Just because Aunt Tillie has been lucky enough to live to be 90 doesn't mean she knows how she did it—and neither does modern medicine. Some people, and they are very much in the minority, manage to ignore high blood pressure, cholesterol, obesity, smoking, and exercise, and get away with it. The real problem is: None of us can be sure we will be Aunt Tillies until we reach her age, and most of us don't make it.

One goal of stroke prevention is to discover how Aunt Tillie has survived, what she has in her body to enable her to outlive almost all her contemporaries, so that we all can be Aunt Tillies. On that day the medical definition of stroke will be archaic, and stroke will have only pleasant meanings, a caress or a bit of good luck. A stroke of bad luck will be a thing of the past.

In the meantime, there is much to be done. Until recently, the stress has been on stroke *rehabilitation* rather than *prevention* and, while we are learning how to prevent stroke, rehabilitation will continue to be important. Through it, the majority of people who survive strokes are able to return to useful lives: It has been estimated that out of every 1,000 stroke victims who survive, 55 percent return to normal lives, requiring some help; and 30 percent, requiring no help. Only 15 percent may be so handicapped that they require hospitalization or total care for the rest of their lives. Rehabilitation, then, important as it is, is after the fact, after the stroke.

What is needed now—and is starting to happen—is more attention to what happens *before* the stroke, in the hope that we may be able to prevent strokes.

Medical research has begun to identify the underlying causes of stroke. Studies such as the Framingham study have scratched the surface in identifying those people who may be stroke-prone. In some measure, we know what can be done to prevent their having a stroke. We have yet to know for certain all of the factors, either alone or in combination, that may lead to stroke. But we do have some good leads. Modification of factors leading to stroke is now feasible.

One of the reasons for this increased attention to stroke prevention is that people are living longer lives, and stroke does tend to strike hardest and more frequently in later years. At the same time, stroke does not respect age any more than it does sex. Children, too, can be victims of stroke, although fortunately this is quite rare.

Preventing stroke, therefore, means answering these questions:

1. How can we better identify stroke-prone individuals?

2. How can we better treat individuals identified as stroke-prone so we can prevent stroke?

3. What can we do to prevent any stroke from happening? When should prevention start? At what age?

Stroke prevention actually starts in your physician's office. When you go to your doctor for a checkup, he is in effect "screening" you. He is determining by his examination whether you are stroke-prone or heart-disease-prone or whether you have cancer, or not. In addition, he already knows your age, sex, and heredity. He knows what work you do, where you live, what your diet consists of, your weight, whether you smoke, whether you exercise, and perhaps what stresses you are under. If you are a female, he knows whether you are taking the "pill."

By his history, physical examination, and laboratory examination, he is looking for:

1. High blood pressure
2. Evidence of heart disease
3. Evidence of diabetes
4. Evidence of gout
5. Evidence of high blood fats or high blood cholesterol

6. Evidence of more red blood cells in the blood than normal

There may be other tests, too (to check for cancer), but all these factors and findings go into what constitutes risk factors in stroke. Some of the factors carry an excessive risk. Some have not been proven to carry excess risk, and other factors may even be protective.

Identifying the Highly Stroke-Prone

If a person has already had a stroke, the factors that contributed to his having Stroke Number One are likely to be present to possibly cause Stroke Number Two. Doing everything to reduce this person's risk factors is necessary to prevent that second stroke.

To begin with, reduction is necessary: Reduction of an elevated blood pressure, reduction in elevated blood fats, and—of course—weight reduction. Besides reduction, other treatment is necessary, such as treatment of assorted medical disorders. We must control existing diabetes, heart disease, gout, and polycythemia (excess red blood cells). Under certain conditions, the attending physician may advocate the use of anticlotting medications. All of this means that even if a person has already had a stroke, his outlook is brighter today in avoiding a second stroke than it was a decade or two ago.

People who have had strokes, then, are considered to be highly stroke-prone. Another category of people considered to be almost as highly stroke-prone are those who have had transient ischemic attacks, since the vast majority of people who have them eventually do suffer strokes—if they are not identified and treated.

These prestroke warnings are temporary episodes that last a few minutes. Usually they go as quickly as they come, so that some people tend to ignore the warnings. They say, "Oh, it was nothing at all, just some weakness or numbness on one side of my body.

Besides, it lasted only a few minutes." A few days or weeks later, the person who says that may have a stroke.

In the future, hopefully such people will not disregard these early warning signals. Hopefully, they will report such transient weakness or numbness or impaired vision or difficulty with speech to their physicians for appropriate evaluation by him.

Other Risk Factors

Preventing stroke or future stroke in these two categories of people, then, is one of the first considerations. But this is only the beginning. Ideally we would like to prevent persons from reaching these high-risk stages. For this reason, investigators must reach even further back into the genesis of those factors that are felt to contribute to stroke.

Hardening of the arteries is felt to be one of the major causes of stroke. The late Dr. Paul Dudley White, the famed heart specialist, wrote recently, "Prevention must become our goal, and our first priority must be atherosclerosis, which has reached epidemic proportions in the United States." He added, "What is required is a widespread change in established habits of overeating, physical lethargy, and heavy smoking—not an easy task."

We must try to learn more about hardening of the arteries and how it affects the arteries of the brain. We know a great deal about how it starts in the aorta; we know a great deal about the coronary arteries and heart disease—but much more needs to be learned. We know far less about how hardening of the arteries starts in the brain and how to assess it and its extent.

Better diagnostic methods are only one side of the hardening of the arteries picture. We also need to know: Are there methods and means by which we can *de*celerate the advances of atherosclerosis in the body? Is it treatable with medications? New drug applications for these purposes are being filed with the Food and Drug Administration (FDA). These drugs may benefit all of us, if they live up to the claims that their advocates make. Until these claims are proven through the use of controlled studies and the drugs have been approved by the FDA, we must wait.

Still, there is hope that in the future we may be able to prevent some of the *damage* of hardening of the arteries, if not hardening of the arteries itself.

Since thrombotic stroke is often related to hardening of the arteries, we must look for ways to prevent thrombosis. Thromboses have been treated with urokinase, a substance that helps dissolve the clot. Of little value in *established* strokes and heart attacks (because the damage is already done), this drug does point the way to further research in this area.

In fact, the use of substances that prevent the initial stages of clotting is the most promising area in the drug spectrum of stroke prevention. Perhaps a medicine as innocuous (or as dangerous) as aspirin will decrease the risks of stroke and heart disease. Carefully controlled studies are needed and are in progress.

High blood pressure we feel sure is a significant warning of a possible hemorrhage or thrombosis. Although recent investigations have indicated that treating high blood pressure disease may reduce the risk of stroke, we still need to know more about *what levels* of high blood pressure need more vigorous treatment. Despite the proven effectiveness of drug therapy, we also need to find better ways of screening large groups of people to find out who has high blood pressure. Once we find these people, we need to know ways of *motivating* them to continue treatment. The high dropout factor in high blood pressure treatment is well known, and until people come to realize that hypertension presently requires a lifetime of treatment, physicians can do little to help prevent stroke due to it.

Obesity is a factor that can and should be eliminated. Most observers agree about the relationship of high blood pressure and obesity, simply because the blood pressure decreases when obesity is corrected.

Although a low-salt diet has been traditional and effective in lowering the blood pressure, newer medicines can accomplish the same result without severe salt restrictions in the diet. The relationship of high blood pressure to salt intake, however, needs further investigation. Suffice it to say that we are presently concerned about the use of salt on foods and that relationship to high blood pressure. This is of considerable importance when we think of all the prepared, convenience and ready-to-use foods that are being offered to the public today. As mentioned earlier, for example, baby foods are salted to adult tastes, not to babies' requirements.

There is another factor in preventing high blood pressure. We must identify as early as possible those children or teen-agers with a tendency toward high blood pressure. We must start treatment before the high blood pressure gets out of hand. These young people may have to be protected from overstrenuous activity in sports, since exercise does temporarily raise blood pressure, and from obesity—in the hope that there will be a minimum need for drug therapy.

Age is another factor in stroke, with the risk of stroke increasing with age. Few people believe we will ever find a fountain of perpetual youth (much as we might wish it), but we do need research into aging and how the process may be retarded. There are as many as 10,000 people 100 years or older in this country who have found some "secret" that most people—including they themselves—don't know. That secret may be as simple as merely enjoying life and its pleasures. It is the quality of life, as well as the longevity, that needs to be improved.

Enjoying life, therefore, may include avoiding stress. We do have tests utilizing our knowledge about stress. Stress electrocardiography is a method of testing for atherosclerosis of the coronary arteries. Although the electrocardiograph may be normal at rest, under excessive exercise or other stress it may be abnormal. Although we have no similar test for stroke, further investigation is needed to enable us to develop a simple stress method, which may pinpoint who is prone to, or will get, a stroke.

Other factors about which we know little and which require more investigation include sex, heredity, race, socioeconomic status, environment or geography, and population density. Present knowledge indicates that women taking oral contraceptives do seem to run a higher risk of stroke, but we need more data to determine whether the increased risk is due entirely to oral contraceptives and whether certain combinations of contraceptive agents may be safer than others.

In addition, while we feel that high blood pressure may run in families, we need more facts. Preventive therapy may also be indicated for blacks, since nonwhite incidence of stroke and high blood pressure is much higher than in whites. We need to know more about whether this is heredity or as a result of environment, diet, or other causes.

Diagnosis and Treatment

It is one thing to identify stroke-prone persons through what we know about high blood pressure and atherosclerosis at the present time. As this knowledge increases, and even before, we must have better ways of diagnosing and treating them. We have made a start. Some of the areas of interest are these:

1. *Methods for measuring the flow of blood to the*

brain have been developed during the past 25 years. However, further research in developing a simple method is needed, a method which can tell us what parts of the brain are receiving adequate amounts of blood and what parts are not receiving adequate blood.

2. *Tomography* of the head is an X-ray technique that uses a narrow beam of X rays to scan a patient's brain in slices or sections about ⅜ inch wide. When computerized, this system is 100 times more sensitive than conventional X-ray pictures of the skull. This technique is performed by the EMI scanner. It opens up a new avenue into the study of the brain. It is presently costly, but it may revolutionize our ability to diagnose disorders of the brain.

3. *Thermography* screens certain arteries in the head (for example, ophthalmic artery), reflecting flow in the internal carotid artery, and branches of the external carotid artery. It focuses on the area of the forehead. Facial thermography measures the heat generated on the face. If the arteries are blocked, the heat given off on that side will be less, and a thermographic picture will show this. Again, this method is expensive. In addition, it is not 100 percent accurate at this point. Nevertheless, it may hold promise for a safe, simple method of diagnosing stroke-prone individuals.

4. The actual *treatment* of stroke needs continued research support. For example, breathing mixtures of carbon dioxide and oxygen has been a traditional form of treatment in some types of stroke, on the basis that it dilates arteries, allowing freer circulation. No adequately controlled studies have been done demonstrating its value. The same holds true for some medications that enjoy traditional use, rather than having a scientific basis. The use of these medications and the use of hyperbaric oxygen chambers (administering oxygen under increased pressure) need further clarification.

In the treatment of brain hemorrhage, more precise studies need to be done to:

1. Find medications that will alleviate spasms of the arteries of the brain
2. Tell us how much to lower the blood pressure of patients with high blood pressure and stroke
3. Find medications that will *promote* clotting in cases of brain hemorrhage more effectively than those presently available
4. Effectively tide a patient over until the determination that surgery will be of help in, for example, removing a congenital malformation or an aneurysm

In searching for *new drugs* and treatment, we may also be looking for new uses for "old" drugs. One that has been found effective in decreasing the clotting ability of blood is an old friend—aspirin.

Aspirin, a remarkably safe drug at low dosages, has been reported to enhance bleeding in patients with some gastrointestinal disorders and in occasional patients after tonsillectomy. It has been felt that some people, such as the patients above, are allergic to aspirin and can suffer profound illness from taking it. Nevertheless, research studies have shown that aspirin, as well as several other drugs, modifies the action of platelet aggregation and stickiness is inhibited—with the process of clotting being inhibited as well.

Platelets are one of the three "solid" elements (cells) of the blood. The other two are the red blood cells and the white blood cells. Thrombus formations (plugs) in our arteries are related to what happens to the platelets in our blood. The part of the thrombus that forms first contains only platelets. Preventing aggregations of platelets seems a possible method of preventing thrombosis. When the wall of an artery is damaged (by atherosclerosis), the platelets congregate and come into contact with supporting connective tissue. Complicated chemical substances are released, which cause clumping of the platelets by making the platelets stickier than usual. The process of coagulation in the artery then proceeds to form the thrombus or plug. Aspirin may prevent this aggregation; this is the rationale for its possible use. But don't run out to replenish your supply of aspirin yet. The work needs more testing and confirmation.

The Future and the Public

Regardless of how much scientists and physicians know and learn, it's of little value unless they can reach the members of the public who can benefit from this knowledge. The American Cancer Society and the American Heart Association have managed to reach many, if not all, of the possible victims of those diseases.

Stroke prevention needs a similar program or programs.

Many physicians agree with Dr. Paul Dudley White that prevention must start with young and middle-aged adults—before it is too late for them. The problem is when, if ever, is it too early?

Autopsies of teen-agers who have died of causes unrelated to cardiovascular disease have found hardening of the coronary arteries. Dr. White, therefore, urges a "Children's Crusade," which was launched at the national annual meeting of the Coronary Care Nurses in 1972. At the same time, he admits that at the present this may be for a minority of children whose families have high blood fats or diabetes, and for those teen-agers whose hearts already show coronary hardening of the arteries.

One key to preventing stroke, then, lies with you—the reader. If any of the stroke-prone factors seem to fit and you are not under treatment, see your physician.

One of the aims of science is to make previous work

obsolete. In the light of new developments and advances, it is hoped that the future will make much of our present knowledge in stroke archaic. New understandings and novel approaches are called for. With your support, the future can be bright in the prevention of atherosclerosis and high blood pressure—and stroke.

CHAPTER XIV

WHO IS DOING WHAT IN STROKE

The studies and the number of medical scientists who have contributed to our knowledge of heart disease and stroke, including what we know about atherosclerosis and hypertension, are legion. Unfortunately, time and space do not permit the acknowledgment of the names of all who serve in this battle for life.

The National Institute of Neurological Disease and Stroke is one of ten institutes comprising the National Institutes of Health. Recently, a commission of twelve leaders in American medicine reported to the director of NINDS on a blueprint for national action against stroke.

A major difficulty is money.

In 1970 the NIH budget for cerebrovascular diseases was $14 million. In addition, the National Heart and Lung Institute devoted some of its resources to stroke-related high blood pressure, atherosclerosis, and clotting problems.

The Congress of the United States in 1972 specified that the National Heart and Lung Institute "shall give special emphasis . . . to atherosclerosis, hypertension, thrombosis, and congenital abnormalities of the blood vessels as causes of stroke . . ."

Much must still be done. *Stroke is the single most costly disease in this country.* It has been estimated to cost $1.2 billion per year, *excluding* the cost of physicians' services and nonhospitalized care.

Here are some other figures, which are cited without editorial comment:

1. Americans spend for jewelry each year—$2 billion.
2. Americans spend for golf courses each year—$3 billion.
3. Americans spent for stroke research in 1972 —$6.8 *million*.

The federal government not only needs to apply more funds to this enormous problem, but the voluntary and private sectors that have traditionally supported research also need to do more.

The American Heart Association has provided leadership in this direction. The AHA Council on Stroke has been organized for providing research and training in cerebrovascular disorders. The National Easter Seal Society for Crippled Children and Adults deals with problems of the handicapped stroke victims. The National Health Education Committee publishes information on stroke. For many years, the Princeton Conferences on Cerebrovascular Diseases have been a source of technical expertise and exchange that have illuminated the darker areas of stroke. The author was one of the founders in 1967 of the Stroke Foundation. This organization needs funds and the voluntary services of those who feel that we all must do more about stroke.

APPENDIX A

GLOSSARY

Aldosterone. See Adrenal Gland.
Adrenal gland. A small but powerful gland sitting on top of each kidney that produces hormones which can cause high blood pressure. Adrenalin (epinephrine) and aldosterone are examples of these hormones.
Amino acids. Building blocks of protein. Combinations of amino acids in connection with one another make a protein.
Aneurysm. Localized weakness in the wall of an artery or vein that produces a bulge in the wall. The bulge is known as an aneurysm.
Aphasia. Inability to express oneself through words.
Apoplexy. See "cerebral hemorrhage."
Artery. The conduit (tube) from the heart, carrying blood that supplies our tissues with oxygen and other nourishment.
Atherosclerosis. Hardening of the arteries, also called arteriosclerosis.

Blood fat. Blood fats include cholesterol, triglycerides, and other substances. The fat generally associated with hardening of the arteries is cholesterol. Fats are normal constituents of the blood and are considered dangerous only when levels become excessive.
Blood pressure. The pressure in the arteries generated by the heart pumping blood. (See systolic and diastolic blood pressure.)
Brain infarction. A type of stroke caused by the death of brain tissue.

Cadmium. A metallic element that can accumulate in the kidneys in experimental hypertension.
Cerebral hemorrhage. Bleeding within the brain as a result

of blood vessels that burst, preventing flow of blood and damaging that part of the brain.

Cerebrovascular. Pertaining to the blood vessels of the brain.

Cholesterol. A blood fat that is found in humans and in all other animals. Its elevation is associated with hardening of the arteries and, as a result, with heart disease and stroke.

Circle of Willis. A "circle" at the base of the brain where the four principal arteries to the brain join before branching off to supply the brain with blood containing oxygen and glucose.

Coarctation of the aorta. A localized narrowing of the main artery of the body, the aorta, which causes high blood pressure in the upper part of the body and low blood pressure in the lower part of the body.

Congenital. Implies a condition that is present at birth.

Diastolic blood pressure. In a blood pressure of 120/80, the lower figure of 80 is the diastolic blood pressure.

Embolic stroke. Stroke caused by clots, which may form on heart valves and travel to the brain.

Embolus. A clot forming in one place, breaking off, and moving through the arteries to a distant place.

Epinephrine. See Adrenal gland.

Essential hypertension. Essential hypertension is synonymous with primary hypertension. In this form of high blood pressure, there is no known cause.

Hard water. Water containing relatively large amounts of magnesium and calcium. Soap used with this water doesn't give many suds.

Hemiplegia. Paralysis or weakness on one half of the body.

Hyperlipidemia. An excessive amount of blood fats.

Hypertension. High blood pressure.

Hemorrhage. Abnormal bleeding. In a brain hemorrhage, a blood vessel ruptures for any number of reasons, causing bleeding within the brain with consequent deprivation of that part of the brain of vital blood and glucose.

Infarction. An area of tissue in an organ that has died. If the death of tissue is in the brain, the infarction is commonly called stroke. A myocardial infarction is death of heart tissue, commonly called a coronary or heart attack.

Intensive care unit. A room especially designed to care for critically ill patients. All the body's vital signs (respiration, heart rate, blood pressure, and electrocardiogram) can be monitored through special electronic equipment.

Ischemia. A lack of oxygen in a particular part of the body.

Ischemic brain disease. Disease of the brain caused by a lack of oxygen. This is commonly caused by hardening of the arteries to the brain.

Ischemic heart disease. Disease of the heart caused by a lack of oxygen. This is commonly caused by hardening of the arteries to the heart.

Lanthanic disease. A disease without symptoms. Examples of lanthanic diseases are early diabetes, tuberculosis, hardening of the arteries, and high blood pressure.

Lesion. An injury or wound. An atherosclerotic lesion is an injury to an artery due to hardening of the arteries.

Lipoprotein. Literally fat-protein. Fat is hooked up to protein in the blood and is carried in the blood as lipoprotein. This, in effect, does for blood fat what homogenization does for milk fat. There are different types of lipoproteins: a very low density, low density, and high density lipoproteins. The density is measured by the size of the particles and different physical properties. Low-density liproproteins are the chief carriers of cholesterol.

Milligram. A thousandth of a gram (abbreviated mg.). A gram equals 1/30th of an ounce.

Monosaturated fat. Peanut and olive oil. These fats have little effect on cholesterol levels in the blood.

Myocardial infarction. A heart attack. See "infarction."

Pheochromocytoma. A tumor of the adrenal gland that causes high blood pressure.

Physiatry. The medical specialty devoted to rehabilitation.

Plaque. A stage of hardening of the arteries. Plaques are formed in the arteries as the result of deposits of fat and other components in the walls of the arteries. They partially obstruct the arteries and can lead to clot formation—thrombosis in the arteries.

Polyunsaturated fat. These are the liquid vegetable fats, such as corn oil, safflower oil, walnut oil, cottonseed oil, and others (except coconut oil). They tend to act in such a way as to lower cholesterol in the blood.

Prudent diet. A diet low in cholesterol and saturated fats.

Renal hypertension. High blood pressure secondary to kidney disease of different types. Glomerulonephritis and pyelonephritis are examples of kidney diseases which can cause high blood pressure.

Saturated fat. Basically, fats and oils of animal origin that tend to elevate blood fats and cholesterol. Coconut oil, while a vegetable oil, is the exception—it, too, is a saturated fat.

Secondary hypertension. High blood pressure due to diseases which can be identified, for example, kidney disease, tumors of the adrenal glands, and coarctation of the aorta.

Soft water. Water containing relatively low amounts of magnesium and calcium. Soap used with this water gives lots of suds.

Stenosis. The narrowing of an artery.

Subarachnoid hemorrhage. Bleeding in between two of the covering layers of the brain that contains the spinal fluid.

Systolic blood pressure. In a blood pressure of 120/80, the upper number of 120 is the systolic blood pressure.

Thrombosis. Blockage or obstruction of an artery, due to a clot in the artery.

Thrombus. The clot blocking or obstructing the artery.

Transient ischemic attack. Warning signs of stroke: A temporary stroke, usually lasting for a few minutes. TIA generally leave no permanent effects; between attacks, a person is completely normal.

Vein. The conduit (tube) going to the heart, carrying blood containing carbon dioxide and waste products from the tissues.

CALORIE AND CHOLESTEROL CONTENT OF COMMON FOODS

Many physicians suggest a limited intake of cholesterol as an aid in reducing the risk of disease due to atherosclerosis. The calorie and cholesterol content of the foods listed here will be of assistance in meal planning.

ABBREVIATIONS USED IN TABLES

Cholesterol Content	H	M	L	0
	High	Medium	Low	None

Servings
aver - average
c - cup
ckd - cooked
gran - granulated
Lg - large
med - medium
sm - small
oz - ounce
sl - slice
sq - square
t - tablespoon
wh - whole

The caloric content for prepared foods in this table was not reduced by special preparation, such as given in the suggested recipes. In addition, while many of the foods do not contain cholesterol, they may contain saturated fat and should be avoided. See chapters III and X for information on saturated fats in different foods.

SEAFOOD

FISH	Serving	Calories	Cholesterol
Bass	4 oz	100	M
Cod	4 oz	100	M
Finnan Haddie	4 oz	125	M
Flounder	4 oz	150	M
Haddock	4 oz	180	M
Hake	4 oz	125	M
Halibut	4 oz	200	M
Herring	4 oz	225	M
Herring, pickled	4 oz	150	M
Mackerel	4 oz	150	M
Perch	4 oz	100	M
Salmon, broiled	4 oz	140	M
Sardines, canned	4	100	M
Salmon, canned	½ c	200	M
Sole	4 oz	125	M
Trout	8 oz	225	M
Tuna, canned	4 oz	125	M

OTHER SEAFOOD			
Abalone	aver	100	M
Caviar	1 t	50	H
Clams, steamed	12	100	H
Clams, fried	2	200	H
Crabs	½ c	65	H
Crabs, Cocktail	½ c	90	H
Lobster	½ c	65	H
Lobster Newburg	aver	350	H
Mussels	12	125	H
Oysters	6 med	50	H
Oysters, fried	6 med	250	H
Scallops	4 oz	90	H
Shrimps, average	10	100	H
Shrimps, canned	4 oz	145	H
Shrimp Creole	aver	175	H
Shrimp, fried	6 med	250	H

LAMB, BEEF, PORK

BEEF			
Brains	6 oz	200	H
Corned	4 oz	250	H
Ground	3 oz	310	H
Heart	3 oz	100	H
Liver, beef	4 oz	150	H

	Serving	Calories	Cholesterol
Liver, calf	4 oz	160	H
Pot Roast	4 oz	250	H
Roast	4 oz	200	H
Steak	4 oz	200	H
Tongue, canned	1 c	250	H
Tongue, fresh	2 sl	100	H
Tripe	4 oz	175	M
VEAL			
Chop	1 med	150	M
Cutlet	4 oz	125	M
Loaf	4 oz	250	M
Roast	4 oz	150	M
Steak	4 oz	250	M
Stew	4 oz	250	M
Sweetbread	4 oz	125	H
LAMB			
Chop, broiled	aver	250	H
Chop, fried	aver	325	H
Kidney	4 oz	150	H
Liver	4 oz	155	H
Roast	4 oz	200	H
Stew	1 c	250	H
Tongue	3 sl	150	H
PORK			
Bacon, strips	3	100	H
Bacon, fat	1 t	50	H
Chop, broiled	aver	225	H
Chop, fried	aver	250	H
Ham, boiled	4 oz	350	H
Ham	1 sl	100	H
Ham, smoked	4 oz	450	H
Kidney	4 oz	130	H
Liver	4 oz	150	H
Loin Roast	1 sl	100	H
Sausage, links	2	150	H
Spareribs	6	250	H
OTHER MEATS			
Bologna	2 oz	125	H
Frankfurter	aver	125	H
Liverwurst	1 sl	75	H
Rabbit	4 oz	175	L
Salami	1 oz	125	H

POULTRY

CHICKEN	Serving	Calories	Cholesterol
A La King	½ c	375	H
Broiled	½ med	200	L
Canned	4 oz	200	L
Creamed	½ c	150	H
Fat	1 t	45	L
Fried	½ med	325	M
Fricassee	4 oz	225	M
Giblets	4 oz	150	H
Livers	4 oz	150	H
Pot Pie	4 oz	350	M
Roast	4 oz	200	L
Salad—no mayonnaise	4 oz	225	L
Stew	½ med	225	L

OTHER POULTRY			
Capon, roast	4 oz	225	L
Duck, roast	4 oz	300	M
Guinea Hen	4 oz	175	L
Goose Fat	1 t	145	L
Goose liver	4 oz	150	H
Goose, roast	4 oz	325	L
Pheasant	4 oz	175	L
Quail, broiled	4 oz	175	M
Squab	1	150	L
Turkey, canned	4 oz	300	L
Turkey, hash	4 oz	175	L
Turkey, roast	4 oz	250	L

BEVERAGES

Ale	8 oz	100	0
Beer, Bock	8 oz	175	0
Beer, Lager	8 oz	110	0
Bourbon	1½ oz	100	0
Brandy	1½ oz	75	0
Cider	1 c	100	0
Chocolate Milk	1 c	225	H
Cocoa, Milk	1 c	350	M
Coffee, Black	1 c	0	0
Fruit Punch	6 oz	150	0
Grapefruit Juice	6 oz	75	0
Ice Cream Soda	1	350	M
Liqueurs	1 oz	80	0
Malted Milk	1	400	H
Manhattan	3½ oz	175	0

	Serving	*Calories*	*Cholesterol*
Martini, Dry	3½ oz	125	0
Orange Juice	6 oz	75	0
Scotch	1½ oz	100	0
Soda drinks	6 oz	75	0
Tea, Black	1 c	0	0
Tomato	6 oz	50	0
Tom Collins	3½ oz	225	0
Vegetable Juices	6 oz	75	0
Whiskey Sour	3½ oz	225	0
Wine, dry	3½ oz	70	0
Wine, sweet	3½ oz	125	0
Pineapple Juice	1 c	125	0

DAIRY PRODUCTS AND EGGS

American Cheese	1 oz	105	H
Bleu Cheese	1 oz	95	H
Butter	1 t	100	H
Buttermilk	1 c	85	M
Camembert	1½ oz	125	M
Cheddar Cheese	1 oz	105	H
Cottage Cheese	½ c	105	L
Cream Cheese	1 oz	105	H
Cream, light	1 t	30	H
Cream, heavy	1 t	50	H
Goat Milk	1 c	165	H
Milk, whole	1 c	165	H
Milk, skim	1 c	85	0
Milk, evaporated	1 c	200	H
Milk, dried skim	1 t	25	0
Parmesan, grated	1 t	25	M
Sour Cream	1 t	50	H
Swiss Cheese	1 oz	100	M
Whipped Cream	1 t	50	H
Yogurt, skim	1 c	115	L

EGGS

Boiled	1 med	70	H
Fried	1 med	100	H
Omelet, butter	2 eggs	185	H
Scrambled	aver	150	H
White only	1 med	15	0
Yolk only	1 med	55	H

VEGETABLES

	Serving	Calories	Cholesterol
Artichokes	1 Lg	95	0
Asparagus	12	25	0
Beans, Baked	1 c	200	0
Beans, Kidney	1 c	225	0
Beans, Lima	1 c	150	0
Beans, Green	1 c	25	0
Beets	1 c	70	0
Broccoli	1 c	45	0
Brussels Sprouts	1 c	60	0
Cabbage, raw	1 c	35	0
Cabbage, cooked	1 c	45	0
Carrots	1 med	25	0
Carrots, cooked	1 c	50	0
Cauliflower	1 c	30	0
Celery	1 stalk	15	0
Corn	1 ear	100	0
Cucumbers	1 aver	20	0
Eggplants	1 c	50	0
Leeks	1 c	40	0
Lentils	1 c	110	0
Lettuce	1 Head	50	0
Mushrooms	1 c	30	0
Onions, cooked	1 Lg	50	0
Peas, cooked	1 c	110	0
Peppers, green	1 Lg	25	0
Potatoes, broil	1 med	125	0
Potatoes, chips	10 med	100	0
Potatoes, Fr. fried	6	100	M
Sauerkraut	1 c	50	0
Soybeans	1 c	200	0
Spinach, boiled	1 c	100	0
Squash, Hubbard	1 c	100	0
Squash, Summer	1 c	35	0
Tomatoes	1 med	25	0
Turnips	1 c	45	0
Yams, Baked	1 aver	200	0
Watercress	1 c	10	0
Zucchini	1 c	45	0

SOUPS

	Serving	Calories	Cholesterol
Beef Bouillon	1 c	25	L
Beef Broth	1 c	35	L
Bean Soup	1 c	225	L
Celery, creamed	1 c	200	M
Chicken	1 c	100	L
Chicken Rice	1 c	125	L
Chili with Beans	½ c	175	M
Clam Chowder	1 c	100	H
Noodle	1 c	125	0
Onion	1 c	100	L
Pea	1 c	140	0
Tomato, plain	1 c	100	0
Vegetable	1 c	100	0

BREADS, CRACKERS, ROLLS, CEREALS, FLOUR, PASTA

BISCUITS

Bkg. Powder	1 Lg	25	0
Buttermilk	1 Lg	110	M
Eng. Muffin	aver	150	L
Shortcake	aver	175	M
Yeast	1 Lg	100	M

BREADS

Bran	1 sl	75	L
Cinnamon	1 sl	200	L
Cornbread	1 sm	200	M
Date, Nut	1 sl	90	M
Egg	1 sl	75	H
French	1 sl	50	0
Gluten	1 sl	75	0
Graham	1 sl	75	0
Protein	1 sl	40	0
Raisin	1 sl	75	0
Rye	1 sl	75	0
White	1 sl	65	0
Wh. Wheat	1 sl	65	0

CRACKERS

Cheese	3 sm	50	H
Graham Lg	1 sq	25	0
Rye, sm	5 sq	50	0
Soda, sm	4 sq	50	0

CEREALS	Serving	Calories	Cholesterol
Bran Flakes	¾ c	100	0
Corn Flakes	1 c	100	0
Corn Grits	1 c	120	M
Cream of Wheat	¾ c	165	L
Oatmeal	1 c	124	0
Rice Flakes	1 c	100	0
FLOURS			
All Purpose	1 c	400	0
Biscuit	½ c	265	L
Buckwheat	1 c	480	0
Corn Meal	1 c	480	0
Corn Starch	1 t	30	0
Soy, med fat	1 c	230	0
Wheat Germ	1 c	400	0
Wh. Wheat	1 c	400	0
PASTA			
Egg Noodles	1 c	105	0
Macaroni	1 c	200	0
Noodles	1 c	150	0
Spaghetti	1 c	220	0
RICE			
Brown	1 c	130	0
Converted	1 c	130	0
White	1 c	200	0
Wild	1 c	110	0
ROLLS			
Bagel	1	110	L
Cinnamon	aver	100	M
Hard	1	100	L
Hot Dog	1	125	0
Plain	1	100	0
Parkerhouse	1	100	M
Popovers	1	75	H
Sweet	1	125	H
OTHERS			
Blintzes	aver	175	H
Pancakes	1 sm	100	M
Muffin	1	125	M
Waffles	1	125	M

FRUITS

FRESH FRUITS	Serving	Calories	Cholesterol
Apples	1 sm	75	0
Apricots	5 med	100	0
Avocado	1 sm	425	M
Banana	1 med	100	0
Blueberries	1 c	80	0
Cantaloupe	½ med	40	0
Cherries, unpitted	1 c	95	0
Dates, pitted	½ c	250	0
Figs	aver	30	0
Fruit Cocktail	½ c	65	0
Grapefruit	½ sm	50	0
Grapes, Concord	1 c	85	0
Grapes, gr. seedless	1 c	90	0
Lemon juice	1 t	4	0
Oranges	1 med	75	0
Peaches	aver	45	0
Pears	aver	95	0
Persimmons	aver	95	0
Pineapples	1 c	75	0
Strawberries	1 c	55	0
Watermelon sl.	1 med	100	0

DRIED FRUIT			
Apricot, halves	3	50	0
Coconut, shredded	2 t	50	M
Figs	aver	50	0
Prunes	4	100	0
Raisins	1 c	430	0

FROZEN FRUITS
One third of 9–10 oz. package

Apricots		100	0
Blueberries		105	0
Boysenberries		95	0
Cherries		110	0
Peaches, sliced		90	0
Raspberries		100	0
Strawberries		115	0

DESSERTS

COOKIES	Serving	Calories	Cholesterol
Brownies	1 sq	50	H
Butter	6 sm	100	H
Chocolate chip	3 sm	65	M
Oatmeal	2 sm	50	M
Vanilla Wafers	3 sm	50	L

OTHERS	Serving	Calories	Cholesterol
Angel Food	aver	100	0
Cheese Cake	1 sm	350	H
Chocolate Cake	aver	250	H
Coffee Cake	aver	150	M
Cup Cake	aver	100	M
Custard	½ c	125	H
Danish Pastry	aver	200	H
Doughnut	aver	150	H
Eclairs	aver	275	H
Fruitcake	1 Lg	250	L
Gelatin, sweet	aver	100	0
Ice Cream, Scoop	1	150	M
Lady Finger	1	25	M
Pie, 1 crust	aver	250	M
Pie, 2 crust	aver	350	M
Pound Cake	aver	200	H
Sherbet, scoop	1	100	M
Sponge Cake	aver	125	M
Sundae, Fancy	aver	400	H
White Cake	aver	200	M

CANDIES AND NUTS

	Serving	Calories	Cholesterol
Caramels	1 med	75	M
Chocolate bar	1 sm	300	H
Chocolate creams	1 med	75	H
Fudge	1 sq	110	L
Hard Candy	1 oz	110	0
Marshmallows	1 Lg	5	0
Almonds	12	100	0
Chestnuts	8	50	0
Filberts	12	100	0
Peanuts	10	100	0
Peanut butter	1 t	100	0
Pecans	8	50	0
Popcorn, butter	1 c	150	M
Walnuts	4	100	0

POTPOURRI

	Serving	Calories	Cholesterol
Brown Sugar	1 t	15	0
Capers	1 t	3	0
Catsup	1 t	25	0
Cranberry Sauce	3 t	100	0
Dill Pickles	aver	15	0
French Dressing	1 t	100	0
Granulated Sugar	1 t	18	0
Honey	1 t	65	0
Jam, Jellies	1 t	50	0
Maple sugar	1 t	18	0
Maple syrup	1 t	60	0
Mayonnaise	1 t	100	M
Molasses	1 t	50	0
Mustard	1 t	10	0
Olives	6 sm	50	0
Olive Oil	1 t	125	0
Tomato Sauce	¼ c	50	0
White Sauce, med.	1 t	25	H

APPENDIX C

REFERENCES

I. Atherosclerosis
1. "The Pathogenesis of Atherosclerosis," by Wissler, Geer, and Kaufman, The Williams & Wilkins Co., Baltimore, 1972
2. "Clinics in Endocrinology and Metabolism," Volume 2, Number 1, W.B. Saunders Co., Ltd., London, Philadelphia, Toronto, March 1973
3. "Atherosclerotic Vascular Disease," Brest & Moyer, Appleton Century Crofts, New York, 1967
4. "Experimental Medicine and Surgery in Primates," Annals of the New York Academy of Sciences, New York, 1969
5. "Atherosclerosis: Recent Advances," Annals of the New York Academy of Sciences, 1968

II. Diet
1. "The Low Fat, Low Cholesterol Diet," by Clara-Beth Young Bond, R.D.; E. Virginia Dobbin, R.D.; Helen F. Gofman, M.D.; Helen C. Jones; and Lenor Lyon, Doubleday, 1971.
2. "Haute Cuisine for Your Heart's Delight," by Carol Cutler, Potter, 1973
3. "Cooking with Fleischmann Egg Beaters," available from Standard Brands
4. "The Prudent Diet," New York City Health Administration, 1973
5. "The American Heart Association Cookbook," edited by Ruthe Eshleman and Mary Winston, McKay, 1973

III. Emotion and Stress
1. "Psychosomatic Medicine," by John H. Nodine, M.D., and John H. Moyer, M.D.; Lea and Febiger, 1962

2. "Noyes' Modern Clinical Psychiatry," L.C. Kolb, M.D., W.B. Saunders, 1968

3. "American Handbook of Psychiatry," Volume I, Silvano Arieti, Editor, Basic Books, Inc., New York, 1969 (Sections on "Alcoholic Addiction and Personality," by I. Zwerling and M. Rosenbaum; "Anxiety States," by I. Portnoy)

IV. High Blood Pressure (Hypertension)

1. "The Silent Disease: Hypertension," by Lawrence Galton, Crown Publishers, Inc., New York, 1973

2. "Hypertension and the Cardiovascular System," Review of Modern Medicine, Ciba

V. Rehabilitation

1. "The Medical Clinics of North America: Rehabilitation," Volume 53, Number 3, W. B. Saunders Co., May, 1969

2. "Handbook of Physical Medicine and Rehabilitation," by Krusen, Kottke, and Ellwood, W.B. Saunders Co., 1971

VI. Smoking

1. Various booklets on how to stop smoking and the dangers of smoking are available from your local American Heart Association, the American Cancer Society, and the Department of Health, Education and Welfare. Two of special interest are listed below:

2. "Helping Smokers Quit," a guide for setting up a kind of smokers anonymous group, available from the American Cancer Society or American Cancer Society, P.O. Box 218, Fairview, N.J. 07022

3. "Smokers Self-Testing Kit" (HEW Publication No. 72-7506), 10 cents, from the Superintendent of Documents, U.S. Government Printing Office, Washington, D.C. 20402

VII. Stroke

1. "Strike Back at Stroke," U.S. Public Health Service Publication No. 546. Superintendent of Documents, U.S. Government Printing Office, Washington, D.C. 20402

2. "The Medical Clinics of North America," Volume 56, Number 6, November, 1972 ("Occlu-

sive Cerebrovascular Disease," by William K. Hass, M.D.)

VIII. Miscellaneous

1. "Therapeutic Exercise," by Sidney Licht, M.D., Editor, Waverly Press Ins., 1965
2. "The Drinking Man," by McClelland, Davis, Kalin, and Wanner, The Free Press, 1972
3. "Platelets and Their Role in Hemostasis," Annals of the New York Academy of Sciences, Volume 201, October 27, 1972
4. "Geochemical Environment in Relation to Health and Disease," Annals of the New York Academy of Sciences, Volume 199, June 28, 1972

INDEX